midas touch

POST-COVID DENTISTRY

by LINKEDIN AND TOWN HALL ACHIEVER OF THE YEAR
EY NOMINEE ENTREPRENEUR OF THE YEAR
GRAND HOMAGE LYS DIVERSITY

Dr BAK NGUYEN, DMD

by DEAN

Dr JULIO CESAR REYNAFARJE, DDS

by TWO TIMES LAUREATE ICOI WORLD CONGRESS TOP PRESENTER
WORLD'S TOP 100 DOCTORS IN DENTISTRY

Dr PAUL OUELLETTE, DDS, MS, ABO, AFAAID

TO ALL DENTISTS LOOKING TO PERFORM IN THE ERA POST-COVID
SCIENCES HASN'T CHANGED BUT THE FACTS HAVE.
NOW MORE THAN EVER, WE NEED TO UPGRADE OUR TOUCH

by Dr BAK NGUYEN
Dr JULIO CESAR REYNAFARJE
& Dr PAUL OUELLETTE

ISBN: 978-1-989536-40-7

ABOUT THE AUTHORS

From Canada, **Dr Bak Nguyen,** Nominee EY Entrepreneur of the year, Grand Homage LYS DIVERSITY, and LinkedIn & TownHall Achiever of the year. Dr Bak is a cosmetic dentist, CEO and founder of Mdex & Co. His company is revolutionizing the dental field. Speaker and motivator, he wrote more than 72 books in 36 months, accumulating many world records (to be officialized).

From Peru: **Dr Julio Reynafarje**, dentist, Dean of the Peruvian Dental Association postgraduate School of continuing Education. Postgraduate professor for more than 15 years, with more than 100 international lectures and with publications in many languages in magazines worldwide, he is also the author of the book Sfumato in Esthetic dentistry and is an active entrepreneur in Medical issues.

From USA: **Dr Paul Ouellette**, DDS, MS, ABO, AFAAID, WORLD TOP 100 DENTISTS, Former Associate Professor Georgia School of Orthodontics and Jacksonville University. A visionary man looking for the future of our profession.

midas touch

POST-COVID DENTISTRY
by Dr BAK NGUYEN
Dr JULIO CESAR REYNAFARJE
& Dr PAUL OUELLETTE

INTRODUCTION

by Dr BAK NGUYEN

This has been an incredible journey, one through the midst of confinement of the **GREAT PAUSE**. Confined home, I met with the greatest minds and spirits of our industries. Together, we formed **THE ALPHAS** and the **INTERNATIONAL DENTAL SUMMIT**.

Within days, we connected, organized and put up 7 world summits in the span of 6 weeks. From coast to coast, from one ocean to the next, we had speakers from 4 different countries: USA, FRANCE, PERU and CANADA.

Our subjects covered from the adoption of new technology, **TELEDENTISTRY** to the safety protocol post-COVID. We've also covered means to resume our dental practice with patients with **THE OUELLETTE INITIATIVE** summit, ways of rebuilding our trust and relevancy with the public and the governments with **AFTERMATH.** We went out there, sharing our competitive edge to our peers with **THE OVERACHIEVERS** summit.

"The age of competition is over.
The time to collaborate and to share
is now the only norm."
Dr Bak Nguyen

No, I am not imposing, just stating the facts. Within that time with **THE ALPHAS**, I put on the table my power, my influence, my strength. Amongst my attributes, the fact that I can write a book within 2 weeks was a big edge to push our message out.

I was on a roll, 62 books within the last 31 months, at the beginning of the confinement. First Dr Eric Lacoste challenged me to fill a void in our financial system, leaving those, most in need aside.

Together, we wrote my 63rd opus, **AFTERMATH,** addressing the issue. Since we are giving a new twist to the message of the United Nations with the **UN GLOBAL COMPACT**, I am still hoping to have a foreword from the UN secretary… wish me luck.

That took 2 weeks. Then, I moved on writing with *my brother from another mother*, Dr Paul Ouellette. **RELEVANCY**, my 64th book became a platform to rally most of **THE ALPHAS** to present their views and perspective to rebuild our profession at the aftermath of COVID-19.

That also took 2 weeks. As I am writing these words, I have in the back of my mind to start editing the manuscript for Amazon print on demand. Oh, so you know, when I said 2 weeks, that meant that the book is ready and available in 51 countries on APPLE BOOKS! That's what I brought to the table.

Surely, **THE ALPHAS** were impressed, some were skeptical, but as the results were following quickly, it became a theme, one setting the pace to the new era post-COVID, an era where everything is about quick reaction and improvisation, keeping our head cold, and our cool.

By the end of **RELEVANCY**, we were talking about the end of the confinement. That did not happen! It is there that an **ALPHA** and friend, Dr Julio Cesar Reynafarje wrote to me, asking if I was open to write another book, days after the launch of my last. How can I ever say no to a friend, left alone an **ALPHA**?

Julio is amongst the first **ALPHAS** who accepted my invitation. From PERU, he brings another perspective of our profession, one beyond borders. A kind heart and generous soul, that's what I kept from our first interview together. And then, I learned to understand who was Dr Julio Cesar Reynafarje.

An entrepreneur and solutions' seeker. In the summit on the **AEROSOLS**, he brought his A-game to share with the world, designs and solutions that could help us resume our practice without too many financial burdens. Creative and safe, with the rigorous mindset of a clinician.

When, I invited Julio to join in as a guest author for **RELEVANCY**. I did not have to ask twice. One message and a few days later, I had my reply. In attachment a beautiful chapter from my friend from South America.

I read his chapter. The soundtrack of FOREST GUMP was playing in the background. His words and the notes were emerging and dancing together as a poem. With the sensitivity of an artist and the precision of a surgeon, Dr Reynafarje was describing the clinical daily of our profession, past, present and future.

He was not lecturing, he shared with wisdom, sensitivity and humility, it was beautiful! Oh, and only then, did he reveal that he was a DEAN in post-doctoral education!

It is my honor and privilege to be joining forces with Dr Reynafarje in **MIDAS TOUCH**, my 65th opus. I may have come up with the title, the structure and my usual impact, but this time, it was Dr Julio who ignited the fire. Joining us, is my great friend and *brother from another mother*, Dr Paul Ouellette.

Together, we cumulate close to 100 years of experience across the American continent, from North to South. I am from Canada, Dr Ouellette is from the USA and moved from one coast to the other, from California to Florida. Dr Julio Reynafarje is the ALPHA dean from PERU.

It is not only the abundance of time that we bring with our cumulated experiences but the diversity in space. It is said that traveling opens the horizon and perspective. Well, this is us, opening up.

Still writing for our peer dentists throughout the world, this time, we are diving in the operation room. Julio wanted a book that will be the memoir of the **ALPHAS SUMMITS**, one with concrete applications in the operation room, the dental chair and most importantly, our way with our patients. The first time he wrote to me was to write a book about **TREATMENT PLANS**.

As we agreed that I will take the lead, even if he ignited the project, I proposed **MIDAS TOUCH**, not just as a title, but as a theme and a tone, to the writing of this book: **TOUCH**. How post-COVID, are we touching our patients, physically and emotionally? How are we touching their lives, their impression and fear?

As we covered in our summits, technology will ease the transition post-COVID, but with technology, great technology, there is also the threat of being replaced. That's why we, Julio, Paul and I, think that now more than ever, we need to emphasize our **TOUCH**, not just thoughts.

"Caught between technological advancements
and COVID-19, our TOUCH will keep our relevancy."
Dr Bak Nguyen

Keeping my role as host, just like in the **INTERNATIONAL SUMMITS**, I will comment and summarize each author, my **ALPHA** friends. I will also be contributing with my own chapters.

It is with great honor that I resume my writing with Dr Julio Cesar Reynafarje and Dr Paul Ouellette.

This is **MIDAS TOUCH**. Welcome to the **ALPHAS**.

Dr BAK NGUYEN

PART I

"HUMAN TOUCH"

by Dr BAK NGUYEN

CHAPTER 1

"SPOIL YOURSELF"

by Dr BAK NGUYEN

Since this is Julio's initiative, I will let myself go and enjoy the ride. After 2 serious books on our collective future, I would like to take this one on a different path. Rest assured, it will still be very relevant and useful.

As this book is more intended for a clinical perspective, I would love to share my story with you, from a son wanting to please his immigrant parents to a fail movie producer to a successful dentist.

Yes, by now, it is no secret anymore, I am simply not cut for dentistry. Even so, I am now leading the charge for the new phase of that industry, and I was doing that even before COVID-19. COVID propelled me to the front page, now that my work is filling the gaps and the voids left by the evolution of our profession.

But how did I became successful in a field that I despise? This is one of those stories, one where you'll be waking in my shoes and sharing my perspective on how to love and be loved in dentistry!

"To spoil yourself is the best way to keep
an open mind on what is to come!"
Dr Bak Nguyen

Please do not take my words out of context! You can spoil yourself because you have proven time and time again that you have the character and the shoulders to bear the consequences and the results. To spoil bears no other meaning than to listen and to love yourself. So do it! Stop rationalizing and dive in, it's for you! It is the daily investment on ourself is mandatory.

In professional terms, we call it continuing education. Self-education, as personal growth gurus name it. So why label it so badly when it comes to taking care of ourselves, of healing and replenishing ourselves? Enjoy, and feel good about it! Be grateful and feed yourself!

"The hunger is good and you will need to fuel yourself before going out there and start giving again!"
Dr Bak Nguyen

Now more than ever, we need to feel good and secure first before we can reassure our patients. Whatever you are feeling, you will spread, with or without awareness, and despite your best intentions. To feel good is the first order of the day!

I know, it will take more than words to convince you that spoiling is good. So here's my story. As you should know, I became a dentist to please my immigrant parents or, to be straight and brutally honest, to buy my ticket out of the constant pressure of having to prove myself.

I went to dental school, had my share of struggle and prevailed as we all did! For my soul to survive the journey, I needed a distraction from the books and the labs.

I also needed to taste my newly found freedom. So I spoiled myself with the production of an independent movie, as a dental full-time student. I was 100% convinced that it would be a walk in the park…

I began a movie production in my first year of dental school. It took everything I had, tested me to my bones. Failures after disasters, after storms, it took us, my friends and myself, 4 intense years to achieve the project, **QUESTION DE PERCEPTION**.

Today, the DNA of **Mdex & Co** is still derived from what I learned directing my first movie: to communicate, connect and market.

To **COMMUNICATE**. As a movie director, one does not speak to express. One speaks to be understood. Even after, all the process of filming, acting, cutting, adding soundtrack and effects, it is all coming down on what the public will feel and understand. That's how I learned to communicate.

Later on, as a dentist, that allowed me to have an edge with my patients. Things are clear, not only to me but more importantly, to them! I did not get that from the get-go, I had to practice and to refine my art of communicating until it became a skill. Today, it has become a state of mind and a second nature.

To do so successfully, we have to learn to listen, to read, both the verbal and non-verbal cues. If you persist in refining the art of communication, you will find that most people aren't as close-minded as you thought. It is then, that we'll stop speaking, stop selling, stop convincing to really start connecting.

To **CONNECT**. We are humans looking to connect every day with each other, with ourself, with God. Wearing a white coat or a scrub usually speeds up the connection process.

"We are in power, we are in authority.
The power to deliver and the authority to serve,
nothing more, and nothing less."
Dr Bak Nguyen

Beyond the white coat and the scrub is also a beating heart. Let them touch that heart and you'll be halfway to the desired outcome! Medical, dental, and nursing schools had hammered hard in us the other half! Trust that part.

They fear the unknown. Feel their fear and, do not address it, do not rationalize it, share it! Yes, share their fear. We are all in it together! As a moviemaker, I learned to share the same boat with my audience.

As a dentist, I even shared control with them. Soon enough, they trusted me to lead them to destination, with ease, often with joy and friendship.

> "Feel! That's the way to connect.
> Share, that's the way to keep
> the connection going."
> **Dr Bak Nguyen**

To **MARKET**. Just master the last two skills and let go. Actually, we need to trust in ourselves enough to open and share widely who we are, deep down.

Not just on an individual level, but constantly, just as we are entrusted to deliver results, we need to be comfortable with our skills and abilities and stop being shy and insecure talking about them.

Actually, don't talk about them, embrace them without holding back and people will feel who you really are and what you stand for!

"We are white coats, we stand
for excellence, for knowledge, for them.
What is it to be shy about?"
Dr Bak Nguyen

As a white coat, we can project confidence or insecurity. To hide, to doubt and to order around, those are insecurities. To Connect, to listen, and to delegate, and you will find joy in going to work each day.

"Renew your trust in yourself and in people,
so age will become wisdom; expertise, nature,
and empowerment. This is a promise."
Dr Bak Nguyen

The easiest way to replenish ourselves is to do it daily. Spoil yourself, do it daily, feeding on those great feelings, those human feelings you've helped generate daily! Take that to the public and the market is yours for the taking!

Listen, feel and share! It is really true what common wisdom says: what does not kill you will make you stronger! And then, it gets easier!

Easier because of our habits, our persistence, our work ethic. These words are widely used in motivational speeches. Believe it or not, I needed a pause to find them, because they were natural things I do without thinking twice. I never thought about labeling the process.

Discipline, I hate! I am a lazy guy, but what I hate even more is to leave things halfway or to bow to defeat. Labeling is not something that will empower anyone, especially when you apply it on yourself.

Trust me, it took me forty years plus, to finally shake down the labels I had such a hard time learning. If it's natural, it won't be that hard! Today, I go for natural, for what feels right. Often, it's way easier!

"If it's natural, it won't be that hard!"
Dr Bak Nguyen

Still not completely convinced? Today, I have a successful practice as a cosmetic dentist. One of the main discipline I use to give to my patients their rightful smile is Invisalign, a computerized orthodontics way to align misaligned teeth without the use of the metallic conventional braces.

On this I have my ALPHA colleague to thank, Dr Robert Boyd who led the democratization of the science of orthodontics some 25 years ago, cutting through all of the red tapes. Even if not all dentists will agree with his works, Dr Boyd contributed to democratizing the art and craft of orthodontic to the mainstream, both the dentists and the public. He showed us another way, that technology can enhance our reach without replacing us. All my thanks, Dr Boyd.

I owe my success to the training, continuous education, and years of experience. But I also owe it to have embraced the novelty, it brought my practice to the next level

Today, I have patients from all around the world coming to me for treatments. Not all of them, but some even travel as far as half the world to be treated. Even those who just need to drive a few miles to be at their appointment will tell you the ease and amazement they experience, learning to smile with confidence, while in the treatment, and, of course, after!

I feel privileged to share that connection with each of them. To see them bloom and grow into their intended selves. Sounds pretty cool?! Straight and brutal honesty will tell you another story.

I started Invisalign because I was bored! I wanted to play with the computer to get closer to the movie industry that I left behind. Invisalign was the only discipline heavily committed to computers and digital technology.

I jumped in headfirst. And I had no love for neither orthodontic nor cosmetic! I simply wanted to play with the computer! Of course, I had to be consequential and took on orthodontic training. I went as far as to learn to treat people with conventional braces, learning the basics of bone's growth pattern, the physiology of bone development and the science of aging. Believe it or not, my main teacher, Dr Richard Litt didn't believe in Invisalign.

Facing my first patient, I was ready to install braces, but my patient wanted the invisible thing and me, I wanted to play with the computer. So we agreed to use Invisalign; in worst-case scenario: I was qualified to finish the case with braces.

That day, I tasted the satisfaction of connecting truly with a patient. She loved me from the beginning, even before seeing any result. She had the insurance that I was there for her.

My honesty didn't sound like insecurity, it was from the heart. A few cases over, I got referrals from colleagues to treat harder and harder cases. Even my instructors at Invisalign were strongly suggesting not to proceed with some of the cases I presented.

Worst case scenario, I was able to apply the conventional orthodontic braces in each of the challenging cases, if the need presented itself. So I went on, with honesty and an open heart to treat my patients.

Today, the first pairs of metal brackets are still brand new, laying somewhere in a draw at my office. My success is reflected every single time I greet my patients, people I now call my friends. They smile and go through life confident and happy! They believed in me as I believed in myself.

It all started because I spoiled myself! I spoiled and I followed up on it! Spoiling myself forced me to go the whole way to master the discipline, to give visible and palpable results, to be part of an evolution pushing the boundaries. I was honest, open and dedicated to following up on my stand!

We have been trained to go the whole way! We have been chosen because we have what it takes to deliver consistently and with excellence, day in and day out! It's our legacy, do it with passion!

Embrace your powers and be generous enough to taste your own medicine. Yes, you are good at your job! Yes, you are contributing to the happiness of others. Why stop there?

"Embrace the vastness, the possibilities
and enjoy your new found freedom!"
Dr Bak Nguyen

It all started because I needed a distraction and spoiled myself. Today, it is part of the wisdom that I am sharing with you. I gave in and followed through. Try it and feel the power! It was right there, in front of you.

Be generous and trust yourself, keep your heart open and give it a try! Spoil yourself! We are strong, we are resilient, we are committed! Don't forget yourself!

This is **MIDAS TOUCH**. Welcome to the **ALPHAS**.

Caught between technological advancements and COVID-19,
our TOUCH will keep our relevancy.

Dr BAK NGUYEN

CHAPTER 2
"THE PEOPLE SKILL"
by Dr BAK NGUYEN

To achieve happiness, both parties have to cross the line together. So, how do we connect? Some of us have a natural ability with people. Some don't. It doesn't matter where you started, the people skill can be learned and mastered.

"People don't like to be there,
that's the truth, and your way in!"
Dr Bak Nguyen

And this is even truer now than ever before, at the aftermath of COVID-19. As a white coat, the matter of connecting is simplified since most of the people we meet on a daily basis would prefer to be somewhere else, anywhere else. Again, that's in the majority of cases, not all of them...

So if you know that they do not want to be there, in your dental chair, you know something to be true, something upon what to build on. Empathize with them and the connection just started on the right path!

For myself, I didn't have to leap pretty far to experience empathy. I just didn't want to be there either! I was "forced" to become a dentist. And then, my regrets and the failure of my Hollywood's dream weren't exactly helping the dental cause.

As I learned to accept my fate as a dentist, I did not try to hide the fact that I never completely fit in as a white coat. But they kept calling me doctor. It forced me to act as such. Today, I thank them for their trust, friendship, and support; they thank me for my professionalism, honesty, and humanity. It was a fair trade!

A strange kind of chemistry, that human side that people didn't expect and the empathy from both parties to share the displeasure of being in the dental chair. So we became friends.

Not with all of them, but with most of them, the first generation of Mdex's members, my personal patients. 20 years later, some have become pretty close and good friends, still patients at Mdex.

I guess what I am trying to say here is, do not hide under your white coat, it is just that, a coat. Be real with your patients, be respectful and start reaching out to them. You can love your profession without being insensitive to the fact that your patients see you as a necessary pain.

"You can't change their expectations,
but you can change their experience."
Dr Bak Nguyen

And that was exactly what I did. To be brutally honest, I didn't do it because I was noble or wise or anything like that. I did it because it made my life easier as it eased my pain and regrets.

In short, the friendship I drew from my patients provided them with a quality of care beyond expectation. To me, their warmth kept me from depression and darkness. As they kept coming in, I was forced to check my own personal problems at the door, to greet them with a smile and my full availability to solve their problems, their needs.

"A smile will go a long way."
Dr Bak Nguyen

This cannot be overlooked. If they don't smile back immediately, keep smiling and they will all respond in kind, sooner or later. And by smiling, I don't mean showing your teeth every time. Be empathetic, read them, and try feeling life from their shoes. That kind of smile will go a long way.

In my experience, with a genuine smile, half of the problem is already solved, the human side. For the other half, trust in your science, that half of the white coats hammered hard into you.

As such, I will share with you a unique experience. A few years ago, I received a patient complaining about her smile. She lost her husband and was through with the grief. It was time for her to get back in the game, as she put it.

She needed to feel younger and prettier, but not too much. She wanted it and wanted it right away! But again, not too much. The insecurity was such that I first declined to treat her. She wasn't ready.

And then, she came back, saying that she went through other consultations and I was her choice. She felt a good vibe with me! I didn't know what to answer... she made her case and convinced me that she was ready for a new smile. I conceded. I can tell you the regrets didn't take long to appear.

Without getting into the details, her insecurities resurfaced the minute I started the treatment. By then, I was stuck to finish the case. I gave her my best. Every single step of the way, I had to justify and regain her trust, the whole treatment through. She knew she was being difficult but, I was the only one she trusted! I didn't listen to these words until much later…

Long story short, she went through the treatment. Only to show up a week later saying that it was too much of a change. Her teeth were too perfect and she couldn't smile because now, she didn't recognize herself... she was both proud and insecure all at once!

It went on for months. Then, she met someone and everything changed, well almost everything... Today she still has an edge but she knows it and apologizes in advance. I was, and still is, the only one that she trusts. Her victories on the dating scene, that was all thanks to me, in her own words. I gave her something she did not expect, an ear when she felt isolated.

Of course, I won't hide that before the great conclusion, we had some good and bad times. But she was never mean, she just needed to be heard. Even if at some point in this case, I would have preferred to never have taken her case. I followed up on my promise and delivered, not just the medical half but also the human half. She got me way out of my comfort zone and forced me to rethink both the boundaries of my sciences and approach.

After that, my career, as a cosmetic dentist, went by itself. I had to sell neither my treatments nor myself.

> "I just needed to listen, identify the need,
> and reformulate their words into
> steps of medicine."
> **Dr Bak Nguyen**

Cosmetic cases or medical cases, everything is now a charm, now that I connected with people on a human level, often at the first consultation. When you have people showing up for treatment, years after their first consultation, you know that there was a real connection!

I cannot tell you that I will go through such a journey again, but it sure lead me to where I am today, in front of you, talking about patients' cares and human touch.

Today, I see her once a while for check-up and follow-up. We are on very good terms. We even laugh about the whole thing. Every time she repeated it: "It was because of my smile! Even when she was testing me, I kept my smile and it felt genuine!" That's how she came to trust me. And then, she did the same on the dating scene, she smiled and kept smiling. A smile will go a long way!

I owe to that smile my cosmetic career! That is also why I remained that committed to my science: cosmetic dentistry. Until that point in my career, I didn't think that I could connect that much with my patients.

It is then that I remembered her exact words, she trusted me, even while she was complaining, she trusted that I could get her to the desired outcome. That trust she gave me, gave her back her life and more. That trust fuelled the beginning of my success as a cosmetic dentist.

I still remember the day that I decided to commit myself completely to cosmetic. That night, I felt so bad that I couldn't sleep. Did I complete a doctorate and years of experience to now care for capricious desires and superficial people? That particular case tested my resolution to the bone, every time I got to the office for months.

But as I gave it my all and my best, I also feed myself with the stories, those success stories of my patients, on how their lives have changed since. Today, I couldn't be happier as a white coat. I feel blessed contributing to the world, a smile at the time. Again, a smile will go a long way. That even inspire me to come up with:

> "Smile and the world will be yours!"
> **Dr Bak Nguyen**

There is not much that you can pour from an empty cup! You must find fulfillment and satisfaction from your work on a daily basis. Feed yourself with your victories and move on. As you've mastered both the science and the human touch, it will get easier!

A smile will go a long way. But a smile, to be true, needs to feed on real happiness, the happiness that comes from your love of truly caring for a difference. Don't spend too much time digging your heart, look in the mirror instead. You are that person! If not, you won't have lasted that long in the profession! We are white coats.

Just as the patient who believed that I saved her life giving her hope (a story in **PROFESSION HEALTH**), this patient gave me credit for her joy. And she, in turn, will spread her joy to those around her and so on and so forth.

That is how we, white coats, are changing the world for the better, a smile and a heart at a time! It slowly grew on me… to write **CHANGING THE WORLD FROM A DENTAL CHAIR**. What a bold statement, one I would have never made if it wasn't from the confidence my patients drove in me.

We are always there, in times of need, on-call, always on duty! Be there, be whole, be happy! Trust in yourself and in your patients, you matter more than the boundaries of your function. Ever heard of the butterfly effect? Well look in the mirror and look in your files!

This is **MIDAS TOUCH**. Welcome to the **ALPHAS**.

Dr BAK NGUYEN

CHAPTER 3

"BOND AND DIFFERENTIATE"

by Dr BAK NGUYEN

Dr Julio Reynafarje wanted this to be the memoirs of the **ALPHAS SUMMITS**. Well, we had a summit titled **THE OVERACHIEVERS**, in which overachievers in the dental field volunteered to share their secrets and edges. That was in good sport.

By the end of that summit, my friend, Dr Eric Lacoste threw me a curveball, all in great spirit. He asked me how do I reconcile the need for health treatments and elective treatments, since I am a cosmetic dentist? Well, I was well prepared to answer most financial questions, but that one, I did not see coming.

At the top of my head, I answered with what came naturally: it made me a better dentist and a better person since I learned to listen to my patients. What was a curved ball allowed me to finish the summit with a homerun.

If we take the time to dig in a little deeper, this is the reasoning:

"A white coat is 50% science and 50% human."
Dr Bak Nguyen

We have spent time and energy mastering our craft and science to the summits of excellence. Today, we can hardly distinguish our expertise from ourselves, this is how dedicated we are! The beauty is that this is normal for us, it is a standard of care in our profession, white coats!

Sometimes, the science can be overwhelming, I share with you the pain and hassle. We all had our fair share of hassle. Post-COVID, we will soon realize that everything we've endured was to better prepare us for what's coming. But no matter the pain, no matter the crisis, people are people and fear is fear. The pain is the same.

Eventually, it all comes together as a whole and ends up making sense. Do you know why it makes sense? Because we are still here to tell the story. That means that we were there to put all the pieces together and solve the puzzle, otherwise, we will have been left behind and forgotten.

It's the human part, harder to grasp. How to establish a human connection wearing a white coat without losing professionalism and, at the same time, being accessible and warm? Some will say that this is an art with a thin edge.

Start with the beginning and readjust on the way. Each patient is unique and we will need to refine, somehow, our approach and our words. The best bet we can make is to master the **art of flexibility** and **adaptation**, quick and effortless adaptation.

"Embrace your liability to make
them into your strength."
Dr Bak Nguyen

After listening to your patients and understanding their needs and desires, the next step is to elaborate a treatment plan, one that will answer all or most of their needs and desires.

You then need to make sure that all parties understand each step and also the relative importance of every single procedure, the whole perspective and the desired outcome.

Reality check, we will also need to offer an alternative course of action to rally the available resources to our cause. It is a process and an evolution, to both, your patients and to yourself.

As your patients are opening themselves to a world of possibilities, you are opening yourself to them. Only from that spirit of trust can we build a successful treatment.

We are white coats, that is our calling and the bond that we share with an elite and dedicated group of people. But now, how do we differentiate ourselves? That's the second step after the affiliation. The need to bond and then, to differentiate are part of the natural instinctive needs described in the pyramid of Maslow*.

*Abraham Maslow is a professor of psychology, father of the hierarchy of needs and among the most cited psychologists of the 20th century.

In contemporary words, how do we sell ourself? We all hate that word, selling. It is what it is. If you want my take on the matter, embrace your liability and make them into strength. Allow me to explain.

As a cosmetic dentist, I am upheld by the highest standard of the profession and, on top of that, I am obliged to keep my patient happy the whole way through the process.

In legal words, if they complain, the disciplinary committee will always hold me responsible until proven otherwise. As an elective aesthetic provider of care, the burden of proof rests upon my shoulders, every time.

In other words, every time that I accept a case, I am liable until completion. They may have a good sense of it without knowing the exact words. So, I embrace the liability as a promise of a standard of care to them! I tell them, upfront, that we are married for the duration of the treatment and, as I am a lazy guy, I just want the least problems to occur.

Problems are just slowing me down! What they have just heard is that all surprises and extra costs are not welcomed. We just bonded! Right there! I said out loud something that was on the back of their minds but hasn't yet formed into distinctive words.

"Give them your heart, you will have
their trust in return."
Dr Bak Nguyen

As I jump on the sword and embrace my liability as a doctor, I gain their trust, giving them the insurance that I will be there until the end, in a good way. That's how, for the last twenty years, I have translated my liability into strength, being a white coat.

I didn't have to differentiate myself by doing anything more than leveraging my integrity. The beauty of it? It didn't cost me anything more than what was already asked of me by the law and ethic committee.

I just presented the facts under a different light, upfront! For now nearly twenty years, it worked like a charm. Of course, we still have to deliver our science to perfection!

"Give them what they need. Tell them what to feed.
Make them feel warm and neat"
Dr Bak Nguyen

We are caregivers, we are the healing hands of nations, we are white coats! We have been given the authority to serve, the science to care, nothing more and nothing less.

As we act as doctors and magicians on a daily basis, telling people what to do. We, sometimes, need to be reminded of our role, to serve.

"Humility is to know that we are there to care and to serve. Confidence is the faith that we have in them, in our hard hammered sciences and in ourselves."
Dr Bak Nguyen

Reminding ourselves that we are servants wearing a white coat will keep us from playing with divine pride and lose footing from the thin edge.

Knowing who we are and feeding on the human success stories derived from our everyday actions will keep our pride in check and elevate our spirit in the perspective of the scope and impact we have on the world.

Make no mistake, more than surviving, we are all looking to find elevation, only, some of us got lost and settle, misunderstanding security for misery... Don't settle, refuse to survive so you can thrive!

"You are more powerful than you think!"
Dr Bak Nguyen

And then, we have to deliver, everything that we've promised. And every time, we do, we deliver. That's the hard hammered science working within us. Be grateful. Trust yourself, trust your senses and do not torture your soul with useless doubts!

We are white coats, we have been chosen, selected, then trained to be up to the task, every day, every time, anywhere! That is who we are! Trust that part!

"As a white coat, be open
and stand your ground."
Dr Bak Nguyen

As you have opened up and listened to their desires, you understood what they wanted and needed. Now it's game time! The field is yours. **Listen** to them, make sure they know that you heard them loud and clear, and **stand your ground**.

Never leave your ground. There can be emotions on the way. You, you were sensitive and human, but we are also white coats, so stand your ground, in science, in medicine.

As soon as the desires and needs are clarified, the science part takes over. You can still be human and gentle, but emotions have no bearing on you for the time of the execution. That's why they came to you in the first place, that's why you are good at what you are doing!

So again, don't second-guess your abilities, it's not a God's complex to know your skills and to have faith in the outcome. All my life, people around me tagged me as arrogant.

As I put my hands in the service of my patients, arrogance became confidence. It happened by itself, overnight. I was still the exact same person. Trust in yourself!

"Be a problem solver
and reverse engineer."
Dr Bak Nguyen

Need I elaborate more on this? You know the job. But if you still want to gain speed and momentum, here's a secret of mine. I start with the end, the outcome. As I know where I need to end up, I reverse engineer the steps to the beginning.

It also has the benefits of narrowing down the alternatives of treatments possible. It's simple math and good logic. You'll need something stable upon what to build, and often, very often, that is the outcome expressed by your patient.

If they decided to change the plan, they know that they have also changed the outcome! Trust yourself and trust them! Just for the sake of happiness, be crystal clear about that!

The world owes you much of its joy and life since you are the caregivers, the magicians, the healing hands of nations! Yes, we are strong, we are resilient, we are committed! It is possible to be both, science and heart, medical and human, wise and kind. We are white coats.

Trust in yourself and trust your patients. You are more powerful than you think, just take the time to pause and contemplate the result of your actions in the world. It is called life and joy. And from their fulfillment, comes yours.

Them first, and then, you. That's your nobility, to have put them before you. But you come right after. Do not forget yourself! Allow yourself to be whole, to know your heart, to empower your mind, to trust your guts.

This is **MIDAS TOUCH**. Welcome to the **ALPHAS**.

Dr BAK NGUYEN

50

CHAPTER 4

"HARMONY"

by Dr BAK NGUYEN

I am sure that you didn't expect how unconventional this book will turn out to be! This is me being close and personal. Actually, I truly believe that this is me at my best essence since you can apply philosophy to change human behaviors, theirs and yours.

"We are what we believe.
We believe what we think."
Dr Bak Nguyen

Each at our own pace, we will get through with our quest. As soon as you'll experience your whole, a new kind of happiness will start drafting, one that will last, day after day, one that will serve as your baseline no matter the conditions.

You will start flying high with both wings stretched in the skies, with confidence, with ease. You are whole. And your whole can only be accessed combining both your halves: Science and Human.

I will start here by reminding you that you have been selected, carefully chosen, and heavily trained to be champions and heroes.

"Champions and heroes are
average within our ranks!"
Dr Bak Nguyen

Our profession is noble, so are you. Our profession is demanding, strength and resilience, you embody. Our profession is evolving and guess what? You are leading the way! That was true before, now, at the aftermath of COVID, it is do or die. The profession has changed, the expectations have changed, the only question is, have you?

What is next? No one can expect a different outcome if one keeps doing the same thing, over and over again.

"Habit does not go with evolution.
Comfort does not go with evolution."
Dr Bak Nguyen

In the same line of thoughts, happiness cannot be solely found in habits nor comfort, not to us, white coats. We have been trained to lead the way, to always seek for more, to seek better. In the **OVERACHIEVERS SUMMIT**, Dr Nach Daniel said that we are not overachievers, we are over seekers. Well, we are all over seekers, therefore, we are all overachievers. We are white coats.

From the type of personalities, our profession includes the type A and the others. One is driven with optimism while the others are fuelled by insecurity. Both will do the job, but why is it a world of difference between them?

There is hope, even if most of us are born with the traits, the experience and training will eventually triumph over the insecurity. Keep over seeking! This is not about labeling nor differentiating, the type A and the others are about self-diagnosis and evolution.

Whatever you feel is what you will spread. This is why it is so important for each of us to find our footing, our happiness first. This is the only way to an human touch.

I said time and time again, a half cannot be happy, only a whole can last in happiness. Insecurity is the common symptom from a half. Science alone cannot bring happiness, why not completely silence the insecurity it bears?

"The discovery of science is bathed with doubt,
but not its application. Remember, we are white coats."
Dr Bak Nguyen

Getting back to the **OVERACHIEVER SUMMIT**, the homerun I scored at the end was not only about listening to our patients but also to have the humility to accept that perfection is a lie! A big fat lie! If one wants to achieve and succeed, it is not perfection one should seek, but harmony! And with harmony comes the flexibility to readjust the parameters on the way. That's **harmony**.

Well, guess what? Happiness cannot be obtained through perfection either. Have you ever experienced such feeling, one where you should be so happy standing on a win, and yet, you felt so alone? Perfection does that to your soul!

To be happy, we must be human. That was the missing key. And to grow the human half, as white coats, it is almost too simple: open your heart and your eyes to the consequences of your daily work.

See the good you are bringing to the world, see the ramifications of your emotional investments in the grand scheme of things. We are trained to do good. We are bonded to be good. Simply take the time to appreciate all the good you brought into the world, as a white coat.

In India, we are called healers, a title second only to the Gods! Don't brag. Be proud of your accomplishments. This is from my friend, senior professor of periodontology, Preetinder Singh!

As you feel the warmth of the rising sun on your face, you will gain more and more strength as a person, as a human.

"Insecurity, like moisture, can only exist where there is shadow.
Not within the light of the sun!"
Dr Bak Nguyen

They will leave insecurity behind. It will be natural like it was always meant to be. Like the snow melting and uncovering the land, the flowers will bloom and the colors will paint the canvas. It is beautiful, it is optimistic.

That's your whole, and as you know how to get there, you will never want to let the feeling go. Keep the moisture at bay, leave the cocoon and you will have found your true self! You are now whole.

Powerful is whole.
Happy is whole.
Strong is whole.

And what could you do with your new-found powers? Exactly what you did before, but now, with ease, with more kindness because now, you can really completely forget about yourself to dive into the task, in the care. Insecurity was the daily reminder of one's half identity. With that gone, we are whole, so we need not be reminded of who we aren't anymore.

"To be selfless, one needs to be whole first."
Dr Bak Nguyen

Usually, this kind of talk is pretty difficult, often impossible with a large crowd. People are from such different walks of life and horizons that it is just not possible to guide them to find their whole within a short and concise way.

We are all white coats, we share the same DNA, we are from the same selection, the same training, the same challenges, the same goals, at least from our half science part. We can all make it to the other side and to be whole. We are white coats, to us, it is a **matter of choice, not of merit**.

Trust in you and find your whole. Open your heart and touch the power waiting for you, just at your feet. Power? Is it real power some might ask? Actually, the power is not out there, the power is within you. It has always been there.

Once whole, you now have the key to unlock and unleash your true self, your inner powers. To each, his powers, to each, his destiny.

Mine was speed. The ease to see through the process and to execute it with precision and speed. I could do so with nothing but the insurance that I will achieve my goals.

I have nothing on my mind nor on my heart to slow me down, to doubt about. I know that I am working for the better good of my patient, that's enough for me to keep moving forward.

I trust in the science and skills that I have received as a legacy. Every day, I honor them with myself, my whole. And happiness in all of this?

"Pain is physical, fear is mental."
Dr Bak Nguyen

More than physical pain, the apprehension and fear can eat up an entire soul if time is abundant. Be kind and human enough to understand what they are going through. Ease their pain, both mentally and physically. Speed will do just that, speed empowering your white coat!

"Being whole will lead to selflessness.
Selflessness will lead to lightness
and lightness is speed!"
Dr Bak Nguyen

My assistant will tell you: once whole, as we operate, even time seems to blend to our pace. I do not work faster, time is slowing down. I even have more time to be kind and gentle.

To care, really, deeply. You wanted to cheat time, be whole! You wanted to please and surprise your patient, be whole, selfless and light.

They will love you for it. Grow from their love, heal from their successes. Remember each face and hope from each smile you drew. Your most prized possession is your credibility. Surprise them with ease and speed and your credibility will grow. Beat their expectations and the pain will fade away!

It all boils down to insecurity. Insecurity can be tainted and be overcome, by being whole, by being selfless, by being happy.

We have worked too hard to fail happiness. Especially when it's waiting at your feet. Harmony is the key.

Embrace yourself to embrace your patients. Be happy to spread happiness. Be whole to be selfless. We were born type A or we have reached type A, the difference does not matter. Just know that there is no reason to stay stuck. Life does not have to be that hard.

You owe it to yourself and to your patients to be whole and happy. We are the caregivers, we are the magicians, we are the healing hands of nations. We are white coats! The universe shall shine from our passion and love!

This is **MIDAS TOUCH**. Welcome to the **ALPHAS**.

Dr BAK NGUYEN

CHAPTER 5

"HOPE"

by Dr BAK NGUYEN

Can dentistry be philosophical? To that question, I think that we must, since we have such a void of leadership and vision to fill. Please, I am not insulting anyone, our relevancy went from 100% to 3% within the COVID crisis. It is time that we do more than look at the teeth. We need to look at the whole, not just the teeth.

As I said before, more than ever, our patients need us to reassure and to heal them. The first virus we are treating should be **fear**, and then we shall address the illness. Understand that, master that, and all of your treatment plans will have a chance to change someone's life for the better.

I don't know about you, but to me, that's relevancy. And what is left on the table, once fear has been chase away? Hope, not facts, **hope**.

To enjoy the fruit of your efforts and devotion, we need to be open to the possibilities, to accept that some things new could happen to surprise us. Just like you have embraced the possibility of life, of healing, the people and the world to the best of your abilities.

Accept the offerings from the universe with the same passion and strength you showed, refusing to kneel in front of illness and death. That's not playing God, that's hope, the power to be human. That's the power we have as white coats.

As a white coat, we are healers. If all we seek was based solely on facts, we could easily be replaced by machines, precise, and consistent. But that's not how medicine works, that's not how dentistry works.

We all learned the placebo effect back on the school benches. Well, it works both ways. If you think that you are healing, you are. If you think that you are sick, well, you are too!

These are soft facts we all need to address even within the cold factual world of medicine and proof. Put differently, treat a patient without the power of hope and you are running uphill and against the wind!

The warmth you have, no machine can ever replace, those are hope and trust. That human touch is what helps the healing process, one bathed in hope.

If we keep pushing, the light will show
If we keep digging, the water will flow
If we keep hoping, we will grow
That's the power of humanity, to hope.

To hope is to be optimistic, to believe the best in the world and its possibilities. Some of us are born optimistic, some will demand more answers before believing. That's okay.

To build a great and lasting world, we need both, the optimistic and the cautious. But being optimistic doesn't mean to hope and wait. Nor being cautious means to be close minded and hide behind protocols and safety.

The body is not purely mechanics and the systems, half of them are the beliefs and the hormones responding to such beliefs. That, we all knew, we are white coats.

"We do and hope for the best."
Dr Bak Nguyen

So hope and fear are no positive thinking nor BS. They are responsible for the hormonal response of the body to the treatments, drugs and all that you'll be prescribing. Never forget that your science and white coat were only half of the DR title you are wearing.

Hope is a theme, with similar effects as chords in a song. Nothing will just happen by itself. Rejecting the possibilities will just narrow down your chances of success. There is a world between being right and not being wrong.

Don't get me wrong, I love to be right, but I will humbly accept to not be wrong too. In that difference lays the scope of possibilities, possibilities available only to those with open minds and hearts. Look at it the way you want, it is still the best course of action for Humanity. And to be happy, we need to be humans.

"Do, hope and welcome the possibilities."
Dr Bak Nguyen

We are white coats, half science and half human. Our human's half will hope while our science's half will be more cautious and demand a sure answer. We are both. To be whole, white coats, we do not need to choose between science and humanity nor between hope and caution, we need to embrace hope with all our heart, and give it our best shot with all that we are, and all that we know. God will do his part, as we fulfilled ours.

Do no harm. To stop believing, to give up on hope, we are harming ourselves as we have given up on the chances of life and, by extension, choose to leave our patients with nothing but the lack of power to make a difference.

We may not save everyone, but with hope, we won't have condemned anyone either. Our job was to give it our best shot, every single time.

"As caregivers, we have the obligation
to believe first."
Dr Bak Nguyen

The body reacts to the mind and morale. Some will disregard these facts but they are real variables of the power of hope. And that was just the mind. Imagine if the heart joins in too?

To believe is a powerful thing. What I am asking you, is to believe in yourself and to be humble enough to stay open to the possibilities, to be right and also to not be wrong.

"We have worked too hard to fail happiness,
blinded by our desire to be right."
Dr Bak Nguyen

Be, do and hope. To be whole, we needed to open our hearts to see the ramifications of our impact on the world. To be whole and useful to the fullest of our capabilities, we need to believe that beyond what we know, there is more, that beyond what we see, there is better, there are worlds to be discovered.

No heart and no mind can grow without the hope of finding more from the journey. The end will come, eventually. But in the meantime, the journey is worth the walk!

Only when we have understood that
We will have mastered the healing
Of both the body and the spirit
Only then, we could be whole and selfless
Only then, we will be truly happy

This is **MIDAS TOUCH**. Welcome to the **ALPHAS**.

Dr BAK NGUYEN

CHAPTER 6
"MENTORS"
by Dr BAK NGUYEN

White is our color. We are white coats. We are always there, in times of need, on-call, always on duty! We give the best of ourselves, out there on a daily basis and we do not have the right for failure, even if the odds are all stack against us. In any other field, this is called being a champion. We, we call it average.

We give it our best, every day, always putting the needs of others before our own. Often, we even forget that we had needs until the pain has reached an advanced stage... In any other field, this is the mark of heroes. Often the selflessness was punctual, not daily. Within our ranks, on a daily exercise, we call it, average.

To top it, we do not talk about it. Humility, in all cultures across time and space, is a sign of nobility, of goodness, of greatness. We, we call it doing our job! Remember, you've been selected amongst the bests, chosen again and again to reach the pinnacle, the next level, heavily trained to serve humanity with your science.

We are part of the world's elite forces to do good, to save, not only the day but also to carry the hope from the ground up, one life at a time.

Take a moment, close your eyes, and feel the nobility and greatness of your character. You are a true champion. You have the heart of a hero! Humility doesn't mean to think less about yourself. We are strong, we are resilient, we are committed!

Facing the odds, we do not back down, even alone, we will fight until the end. We are white coats!

"We are on our own
and we will stand tall!"
Dr Bak Nguyen

This is who we are, white coats. This is how we are built. Standing on our own to serve our pledge against the odds. You can be proud, you need to be proud, but keep pride at bay.

"You might be on your own,
but you do not have to be alone!"
Dr Bak Nguyen

Dentistry with a human touch. Is that even possible? By now, you know my style, I don't lecture. There is nothing I hate more than someone talking down on me and telling how I should live my life. Even if I've written 64 books until now, I am not lecturing, I am sharing.

The last time I was on air and exchanging with an **ALPHA** and **OVERACHIEVER**, Dr Jeremy Krell who is involved in 12 companies on top of practicing as a general dentist, he thanked me for the interview I offered him.

He thanked me and my fans to have given him the chance to talk about his endeavors. Well, I reply: "I have no fans. I only have friends and peers." On that, we laughed and greeted each other.

" Friends and peers!"
Dr Bak Nguyen

I've been the same person most of my life. Sure, I may have evolved, but the older I get, the more I let go of what Conformity and Society drilled into me. I believe in connecting, in sharing and evolving from the differences.

It is with that spirit that I successfully attracted many people to me, great minds and spirits. I won't be here talking about dentistry if I wasn't successful. Well, I would have never succeeded if my patients did not trust me.

For some reason, there were drawn to trust me before the treatment… after, they loved me even more, because I prove them right!

I know that we are not all born equal. Some will evolve more than others. The birth, we did not choose, but the evolution, we each have a saying, a choice. That's choice is what I believe in. On the same line of thoughts, I spent 18 months saying yes to everything, just to reset my mind. Guess what? It worked!

What I am trying to say is that we attract what we are. And since we are what we believe, we end up attracting what we believe! How cool is that? Sure, not every attraction will lead to a success, but in a bigger perspective, we will have gained much more than we lost.

"Don't judge anyone,
even if you think you know."
Dr Bak Nguyen

This is seriously the hardest part, to be right about someone… and to keep that frame of mine not to judge the next person coming. Haven't I told you that I am a multiple world records contender on the number of books written and its pace? Well, that would never have happened if it wasn't because I trusted a crazy mind aiming for the moon.

What he was saying was just crazy, but he believed in it passionately. I could have been skeptical, but since I was in my **YESMAN** challenge, I refrained myself from judging. Well, that person never delivered on his promises, although, his crazy ideas propelled me to start writing. Today, I owe him my awakening as an author.

You wanted proof about the **POWER OF OPENNESS**? Look at my track record. You need more? How about my success as a dentist even if I hated my profession? I owe my success to my patients, but there is more. I owe my love to this profession (one I hate) thanks to the mentors I met on my way. I wasn't lonely!

> "Kindness attracts kindness, success attracts success, everything started with attraction… and attraction only works when one opens up."
> **Dr Bak Nguyen**

Don't go through it alone, it's not worth it. We are surrounded but so often we feel isolated. Rest assured, it happens to the best amongst us. This is the trait of champions, of heroes.

The loneliness and isolation are the results of the intensity of our focus. To tunnel vision on the task at hand and to reach the goal is no obsession. It is our brand, our character.

We are so dedicated that it becomes harder and harder to remove those glasses and to look at the world with a normal and wide vision. This is our fate, white coats, the price for excellence and consistency. It doesn't have to be, but too often, that was the case.

We can break the curse anytime and in numbers of ways. Again, each will have a price attached to it. Efficiency, limitations and impact are the kind of trade-off needed to break the curse. But how about being paid instead?

What if to break the curse, we'll get paid instead of paying a high price? No, I am not kidding you, what if we can get paid to break the curse?

Open your heart and look into your memories, you will remember one or two people that you met on your journey who lent you a hand to ease your learning curve. They have a generous smile, a look that welcomes the warmth and the wealth of human kindness.

They lent you a hand and opened their hearts to you. They are mentors. To you, that's was a stroke of luck to find such kindness. To them, you were the hope of a better tomorrow.

"Once in a while, we can truly connect
with another soul and dance in synergy."
Dr Bak Nguyen

It's maybe time now to look for synergy again. You can look for a mentor, but that's not the way it works. A mentor will come to you when you are ready. You, find a protege, one to mentor, and give back the generosity that you've received.

Synergy works both ways! Even if you never had the chance to have a mentor, do it! Mentor someone, and you will have broken the curse of isolation!

In my life, I had the chance and privilege to meet several gentle and great souls who opened their hearts to me. Dr Roger Bourcier was the first gentleman dentist who showed me the humanity and nobility of our profession.

Often without even saying a word, he inspired me to give my best, to go beyond myself to deliver care, to deliver happiness. I met with him at the time of my failure to launch from Hollywood.

He helped me heal my wounds by showing me the hope and the light of caring for others, as a dentist. He showed me that it was possible to truly connect with those under our dental cares.

"He gave me a taste of their love
and I became a believer!"
Dr Bak Nguyen

It wasn't naivety anymore, I tasted it! Dr Bourcier gave me the hope that good is truly good, that what we do can matter beyond our science and medicine.

If I have truly succeeded as a white coat and find the way to my whole, it is thanks to a gentleman dentist with a huge heart, Dr Bourcier.

Even today, I sometimes can hear him sing from the chair next to mine. Even if he retired, he never really left Mdex, never really left my side.

As my evolution continues, I met with Dr Kien Quan Diec who reminded me of my childhood's passion for finance. Like a father figure, he took such pride to show me the numbers, showed me how my skills set as a white coat can easily transcend into other fields and greatly reduced the price of the entry ticket.

Strange thing, as we connected on finance, he taught me philosophy and grace, generosity and gratitude. We had such fun together and time was never enough! If I am that strong today, I thank Dr Diec, the wise doctor.

I kept my mind and heart opened and continued on my journey, it was getting better and better. Fate put on my path Dr Mohamed Benkhalifa. A great mind who cracked my skull open to allow real growth into my soul.

If I have both the courage and the words to talk with you today, Dr Benkhalifa made it happen. If was brutal, it was gentle, it was unique to feel the hand of a big brother slapping the back of your head and daring you to challenge yourself again and again.

More than a mentor, he became a friend, a coach, a confidant. To this day, he still is! If I truly understood the meaning of power and influence and how to apply them for a better tomorrow, it is thanks to the generosity and wisdom of Dr Benkhalifa.

And still, the journey continues. Opened, loved, wiser, I apply myself to life and hope for the best. As I played music to reconnect from time to time with the nobility and sensitivity of my soul, I had the privilege to share that passion with Dr Jean De Serres.

A leader, an artist, a visionary with whom I shared thoughts and songs, with whom friendship was more important than ambition but also with whom my confidence grew exponentially.

From a dreamer to a driver and a magician, Dr De Serres is the friend that you'll never want to lose; for his warmth, for his counsel, for his empowerment. And we have such fun together! Time stopped every time we are together.

Those were the first 40 years of my life. Then, attraction happened and I felt its power. While opening up and accepting virtually all the opportunities, I met Christian Trudeau, a visionary and builder that I usually read about in books.

Mister Trudeau created billions for a Canadian Bluechip. Well, today, I have the chance to learn with him, from him, to bridge the future of my profession. He is the man who taught me:

> "Leadership attracts leadership."
> **Christian Trudeau**

I pleased myself to repeat that his past is my future.

Then, I met with another great mind, André Chatelain, former first vice-president of one of our big banks in Canada. André led the VISA branch of the bank. By the time of his retirement, he was managing more than 100 billion in volume transactions. 100 billion, I don't even know how many zeroes that is!

Well, he is a friend, although he sits with me as a mentor, those people I respect and love. It is from such wisdom that I am building the new economic model, leading the 2.0 shift in dentistry. How can a dentist have such friendships and mentors? Because I was open and respectful.

If I am of any use to you, my colleagues, my friends, it is thanks to all those great minds who put their hopes and friendship in me. They showed me the way, the power, the wisdom, the generosity that I am sharing with you today.

Their friendship empowered my audacity and kindness. To them, I owe to be grateful and driven. Grateful to live and driven for a better tomorrow for all of us. We are all in this together as a whole, as one collective unit!

"Don't go through it alone, you won't last."
Dr Bak Nguyen

We have worked too hard to fail happiness. And the way is not as hard as you think. Give it your best and keep your hearts open for the rewards.

Give and you shall receive,
If you choose so.
Give and you will grow,
If you allow yourself to do so.

School and education gave me standing and science, my white coat. My patients and mentors gave me purpose and hope, honor and dignity. That's the way to my whole, that's how I contribute to spreading happiness into the world. Thank you, thank you and thank you.

Give, Be grateful and Grow. This is the recipe of Happiness of my great friend Anil Gupta. Well, that's a working recipe! Give it a try, an honest one!

To be happy, one must be human first. To be human, we need to bond and to share. That's life at its best. Be there, be whole, be happy! And once happy, your touch is magical!

This is **MIDAS TOUCH**. Welcome to the **ALPHAS**.

Dr BAK NGUYEN

CHAPTER 7
"REPLENISHMENT"
by Dr BAK NGUYEN

By now, you know where I stand. I am good because I believe. I am kind because I am open to listen, I am relevant because I refuse the lies of perfection and seek harmony instead.

When Julio proposed the idea of writing a book to help our peers on a clinical level, I proposed **TOUCH** as the main theme. My **TOUCH** is the human touch, one that is real and warm.

The joy and magic I deliver to my patients made my confidence and my influence. That magic was from within because I was happy and I spread happiness!

Think of that for a moment, can someone be happy and insecure at the same time? That's impossible on most metrics and parameters. No one can be happy while insecure. But then, on what are we building our security? From perfection and norms? When those reach their limits, it is where we fall! We all saw our relevancy fall to 3% in the COVID crisis. That's a hard fact.

So yes, if you want to succeed as a dentist and last for the long term, if you are looking to genuinely connect with your patient to better serve them, you need to inspire confidence and trust, without sounding arrogant. Our training and licenses gave us a minimum threshold to start from.

"The surgical skills and the technics are only half of the equation. The other half starts with happiness."
Dr Bak Nguyen

We are everything but average. Champions, heroes and humble, we are white coats. Sometimes after an exhausting day out there, keeping the fight up and defying the odds once again, we go home just plain empty.

One needs to recuperate and rejuvenate, and that takes time. But once every while, a note comes through the mail, a personal letter sharing words from one's heart telling the story of how we touched their life. That note, those words, these are the reminders of who we really are.

"To most, the future is the only key,
the past holds no hope."
Dr Bak Nguyen

To us, white coats, it is not completely true. It wasn't at our past that we looked at, but from our past, someone else's future. Hope is the future, and hope, we, white coats, can find from our past. This is why the key to be whole rests upon a choice, not conditional on new merit.

"We have already given!
Now we need to learn to receive."
Dr Bak Nguyen

Words from one honest heart can go a long way. It will fuel hope and ignite passion. Honest words can also bring walls down and heal wounds. Those aren't lines for a novel but the fabric of our inspiration. Open your heart to the possibilities, the adventures and the gratitude, and the words will either flow in or flow out. Either way, you are alive!

"We have too much to achieve to be busy
and ignore our own replenishment
and rejuvenation."
Dr Bak Nguyen

Today was one of these days. A day where I opened my heart as any other day and gave it my best. I finished the day and the week completely depleted, I barely had the energy to finish my late meal before crumbling down on the couch.

I was in for a thick and dreamless night's sleep, or so I thought. Less than forty minutes later, I was pulled out from cosmic darkness by my vibrating smartphone: I've just received a text.

I first just want to silence it and return to my comatose stage. But the phone kept vibrating. So I got up and opened the text. Words, a lot of words.

A page blackened by words was loading in front of my sleepy eyes. I don't know what pushed me, but I started reading. A word, a line, a paragraph. Soon enough, I understood the meaning of the words and the depth of human emotions imprinted in them.

I was moved as the words pull me from my fatigue. It took me a few minutes to regain all my senses. As I got through the testimonials of gratitude from an honest heart, I was revived by a wave of celestial and positive energy. I could see the vibe coming out of the words; dancing, and flooding the atmosphere as they were changing colors.

It was a thank you note from a colleague I helped. She was a professor of dentistry in Eastern Europe, then, she moved to Canada. For years, she tried to regain her credentials without much success. From her own words, I was the first one welcoming her as a peer.

I found ways to legally gave her back her title and dignity. I did it because I fell for her, telling myself how I would wish to be treated if the positions were reversed. As I was kind to her, she opened up and shared stories of abuse and how people are taking leisure to point out her misfortune.

She migrated to escape war! That shouldn't take anything away from who she is and her competence as a professor and professional. What started as a natural gesture of help grew in intensity as I fell her frustration from the stories of abuse…

I am a man of solutions. I did not have the authority to give her her license to practice, but I have the means to give her a platform on which, her past and future can aligned. I can legally give her back her credentials. That moved her to her core.

Reading her thank you note, I enjoyed a moment where time stood still. In the middle of the night, I took my phone and started writing, sharing with you those magical thoughts. To write, I needed to fuel from somewhere, and my resources were completely depleted.

And then, those words came in and the light went up again, suddenly, at full intensity. This is what it means to be whole! This is how to find the key to unlock the power within you. Some times words will do. Some times a hug will ignite the fire. Some other times, a simple but honest look will reboot your mind.

Always, from an honest heart, the energy will flow and create synergy. From there, you can pour passion and results. You are reading the results as we speak.

This chapter was never planned for, nor written in any timely fashion. From the comatose stage of my heavy sleep to the awakening of all my senses, from depleted to shining through, this is the **POWER OF HOPE**, the power of words.

"Words from an honest heart
will revive and grow you."
Dr Bak Nguyen

Have a taste of the human half, of what it bears, and you will be asking for more pretty soon! As Dr Bourcier gave me a glimpse of the love from his patients, I, here, give you a taste of the gratitude and the impact.

Both the size of our hearts and the power of our brains have passed the tests, again and again. We are champions, heroes and humble! We are white coats.

You wanted to know how do I write so many books? Because I find my inspiration from the people I connect with. Some people will have a bolder story, some will have a shorter one, but they all carry a story, one you can share.

You might not write novels, but you are touching lives! Yes, we are changing the world, a smile at a time! Never forget that! You owe it to yourself and to the people whom we serve to stay open to the synergy of connections.

To be happy, one needs to be human, to be happy, one needs to be whole! Once whole, we can finally be selfless. A magical human touch starts with a happy heart.

"True beauty blossoms from profound happiness!"
Dr Bak Nguyen

Enjoy the beauty you've brought into this world. From the happiness that you've spread, flowers are now blossoming, causing more laughs and joy. If you want to be an overachiever, I gave you the source of my inspiration: to genuinely share. Dr Reynafarje and Dr Ouellette can all share with you how much we grew as we shared with one another.

Allow yourself to be whole, every day, allow yourself to feel, share openly, and embrace the day. Do it because you can, not because you care. And then, react to what you've provoked! Empower others, that's your path to happiness, or, to borrow the expression from a fellow **ALPHA**, Dr Agatha Bis, elevate others!

Elevate and share. And then, take the time to feel the story and the victory. Everyone deserves gratitude, even if we do not expect it!

This is **MIDAS TOUCH**. Welcome to the **ALPHAS**.

Dr BAK NGUYEN

CHAPTER 7
"THE MISSING LINK"
by Dr JULIO CESAR REYNAFARJE

I just finished reading the first 7 chapters of this book, I love to read something that I can identify with. Thank you Dr Bak, definitely, in order to shine, there must be fire inside one.

The fire of doing things well is a different fire. It is a fire that is fuelled day by day, with a job well done, with dedication for what we do, with the strength that it will not decay along the way, for the desire to continue growing, to continue doing things well.

"That Fire is not fuelled by fuel, it is a fire that is created from the first day that we decided to help people with our profession."
Dr Julio Cesar Reynafarje

It is not easy to light it, there are many nights of study, a lot of practice to do the perfect things, many disappointments to overcome, many steps to be climbed with great effort, all that and much more are necessary to generate resilient wills and to **engraved with fire** in the service of other people.

When we started this project, I told Dr Bak that I would like to talk about some clinical procedures, and he immediately accepted. The idea was to talk about our daily work, but from a logical point of view, doing and following the concept that I have always tried to instill in my students: to do things in a simple way.

Sometimes it is difficult to come up with such a basic concept, but it is possible. We just need to turn some things around.

To understand the concept of this book, I am going to tell you a story directly linked to the title of this book. At this moment, it magically gives our journey a very special meaning.

Midas was the King of Phrygia, a reign located in the Middle East, where it caught the attention of ancient Greece for its splendor and wealth.

Greek mythology created the legend that everything he touched turned to gold. King Midas ended his days when his capital was invaded, following the custom of the time, he committed suicide.

For the story I have to tell you this is just a part of it, Midas was the son of Gordias, for whom the capital of Phrygia was called Gordio.

An ancient legend tells that father and son made a very complex knot where the ends were hidden between the spear and the yoke of a chariot, this was well known at the time as the **Gordian knot** because it was impossible to undo. It was believed that the person who would undo the knot will become the Emperor of the entire east.

When Alexander the Great conquered the city in the expansion of his empire, he asked that they take him to see the famous knot. He saw it and took out his sword, with an accurate drive he cut the knot, then said: "It is the same to cut it, than to untie it."

A solution that fulfilled the legend, as Alexander the Great came to be registered in history as the Emperor of Greece and of the entire Middle East. The Midas' story is inadvertently linked to Alexander's story, and the human touch is inadvertently linked to problem-solving in a simple way.

This is the reason why this chapter is called the missing link. This is the point where humanity unites with knowledge, so that both unite to always take care of people's health and well-being.

Now after discovering the fire within you, I want to entertain you with a little of our own, showing you how, following the example of many, we cut the **Gordian knots** that are presented to us every day in our profession. Looking for the simplest an elegant way to each problem.

This is **MIDAS TOUCH**. Welcome to the **ALPHAS**.

Dr BAK NGUYEN

PART II
"THE MATRIX"
by Dr JULIO CESAR REYNAFARJE

CHAPTER 9
"ALWAYS GO TO THE BASICS"
by Dr JULIO CESAR REYNAFARJE

I really like to talk about dentistry, I have done it all my professional life. One of the things I learned in my academic life is that one must be clear and be focused on the issue we are solving, to look for alternatives, all aimed at having a good resolution of the case. But in order to achieve this:

"You must see everything with simplicity, practicality, knowledge and experience."
Dr Julio Cesar Reynafarje

Within these chapters, I want to show you dentistry from another point of view, a human point of view, but with two very important elements. See dentistry wisely to choose the best and with the vision of a child, with the simple and loving gaze and passion for what we do.

When we talk about planning in Dentistry. It is necessary to understand that before planning, we must know what resources we have to to collect: the medical and dental information of the patient, and that, once processed, we can solve our clinical case. The resources we have can be cataloged in documentary facts and clinical facts.

Every time we evaluate a patient, we can not only focus on finding and restorative lesions, but we must also investigate more about the general conditions of the patient.

Although for many clinicians it is not an important step, the documentation of these resources are integrated into the clinical history, which is a medical-legal document and a transcendental phase in daily work. It must be clear and precise and above all, an **element of decision** in the treatment of our patient.

The clinical planning elements are all those analog and digital devices that allow us to carry out our clinical procedures and may be clinical or laboratory in nature, and we all have conceptual components that are the set of techniques and knowledge that will allow us to solve the case that we are planning.

What are the Basic elements?

The basic elements are referring to all those information collection instruments that can be analyzed and ordered, allowing us to solve clinical cases. We should always have as much and as accurate information as possible. The more data, the better the diagnosis. As soon as we receive them, we must classify them correctly.

The basic elements are:
- Documentation
- Clinical

Both the documentation and clinical elements are supported by a conceptual framework that will allow us to take the case to its resolution, considering these primary elements as the directional axis of the development of **treatment strategies**.

Documentation elements

The documentation elements are all those registration instruments that allow us to obtain information that can guide the diagnosis of the patient's illness, disease, or dysfunction.

These Registration Instruments can be cataloged according to their means of obtaining:

- **Direct collection Instruments** are all the information obtained through fluid and directed communication with the patient. It is basically the narration of their discomfort.
- **Indirect collection Instruments** are the information that can be obtained using intermediary recording elements.

These instruments will be registered in the patient's medical history, which is the primary axis of the analysis for the diagnosis and resolution of the clinical case.

When I am reviewing each of these documents in order to improve them, it is very difficult for me to withdraw any of them, since they all help us.

Something of the uttermost importance is the conversation where the patient tells us about his discomfort. It is the first emotional approach between the dentist and his patient. It is where a genuine connection begins between the 2 parties.

I can't stretch it enough, this is an integral part of the healing process! I suggest paying close attention to the patient and not to a piece of paper or a computer screen. This implies accepting it as your own subject.

Questionnaires like the one below are part of this approach, it is one way to guide us and understand them better.

Patients Perception Questionnaire (PPQ)

The **PPQ** is an element of basic documentary and direct collection. This type of diagnostic aid allows us to understand what the patient sees and what he wants to address. It helps to better define his priorities, his expectations, not only to collect the objective information but also to evaluate subjective elements, usually of emotional nature that, in many cases, not covered in general medical history.

The **PPQ** must meet certain requirements in order to be properly evaluated. It should be written in a simple way. Patients do not use technical terms, references must use colloquial language in many cases. For example, instead of using the term gingival, the term gums should be used, it is more understandable for the patient.

The sequence of the questions matters too. It should always start from the major structures to the minor ones. It should start with the facial profile, lips, teeth as a whole, individual teeth, and then, gums. The questions should be oriented taking into account the primary discomfort, then the function, and finally the aesthetics, shape, texture and color.

The evaluation of the **PPQ** must be carried out according to sectors, upper and lower. When we evaluate it, the result must be punctual, clear, and must include the **patient's emotional degree** as high, medium or low risk, in order to include it in the treatment strategy.

Clinical history

Many times, filling a medical history is a headache for many doctors. Some, simply copy a template that may be found on the the internet. This isn't optimal. Two things can happen with this document: The doctor does not finish filling the form because it has a lot of information that is not relevant to his query. Something even sadder may happen, the doctor could miss some important part of the story with a form with a lack of information at its source.

The doctor has to make this document a cornerstone in treatment plan, so it must be done based on his specific requirements, and the information contained therein must be relevant to him, his philosophy and expertise.

Basically and by definition, it is a legal medical-dental document in which all the data can help us make a good diagnosis and subsequently order the procedures that allow us for the establishment of a clinical case resolution strategy.

When we prepare a medical history, it must have the following criteria:

- Reason for consultation and current illness.
- Clinical examination.
- Auxiliary exams.
- Diagnosis and prognosis
- Treatment and evolution.
- Reason for consultation.

Is it important? Yes, it is! Because it allows us to record the main discomfort presented by the patient at the time of the first consultation. We can help the patient with directed questions that allow the patient to be more objective at the time of the consultation.

Clinical examination of the patient

Now we start with what we are trained for, beginning to recognize the pieces of the puzzle to solve. When I talk to my students about how to approach this essential part of the diagnosis, I always tell them that we have to start smoothly, easing the trust and conversation.

Start with the data and analysis of the medical history. It is a great opener and will ignite smoothly the relationship with your patient. People are nervous at the dentist, starting with a conversation takes away that stress.

Once the registration of the above information is completed, we proceed to perform the clinical inspection of the patient, in order to record all the signs and symptoms present at the time of the consultation. You have to do it in an orderly way.

We must always pay attention to the first outstanding clinical element in our patients. You must understand the general data of the evaluation, such as general condition, nutritional status, hydration status, as well as the presence of any distinct sign at the time of the exam.

Vital signs

The evaluation of vital signs is very important, due to the current situation, it is necessary to record the patient's blood pressure, temperature, heart rate and respiratory rate. Know that recording the oxygen saturation in the blood with digital oximeters can help us tremendously down the road. We must bear in mind that the **most important route of contamination** for a person is the **oral cavity**.

Stomatologic exam

This part of the medical history is always the one that is generally complete, but it is necessary to check some elements that sometimes go unnoticed by most. When we do an examination, we have to go from the largest structures to the smallest ones, that allows us to manage in order and to be more meticulous with the diagnosis.

Extraoral Clinical Exam

We have to do a general analysis. The following parameters must be evaluated in the extraoral examination: facial symmetry and facial type (brachifacial, mesofacial or dolichofacial). Let's also evaluate the facial proportions, the type of profile, and of course the vertical dimension of the lower third of the face.

Intraoral Clinical Exam

In the intraoral examination, we must evaluate other factors that directly affect the oral health of the patient. We must evaluate the **Caries Risk**. Always try to do an **Oral Hygiene Index**. It is necessary to carry out a dietary analysis, especially the frequency of consumption of fermented carbohydrates, and always take a look at what the patient's attitude and behavior are regarding oral care.

About hard tissues, usually, an Odontogram is performed. We should always evaluate the occlusion and the Temporo-Mandibular joint function too.

About the soft tissues, don't forget to evaluate the gingival tissue, oral mucosa and tongue. We could complement it with a Periodontogram, smile line and gingiva-tooth relationship (gingival smile).

Auxiliary Exams

The more data we have, the better the diagnosis. Like everything in life, the only way to face a problem is to understand it first, that is why the auxiliary exams are always very useful.

These are all the tests that we can attach that can lead us to a diagnosis and treatment planning, all help is welcomed.

Radiology

We must differentiate two types of digital radiology shots: direct and indirect. Direct shots use a rigid sensor usually connected to a cable through which the information is sent to the memory of the supporting computer.

It is called direct because it does not require any type of scan after exposure to X-rays, but rather the system itself automatically performs the digital process and image acquisition.

In indirect shots, the image is taken in a conventional way on a photostimulable phosphoric sensor, and can then be digitally scanned. Both systems work well, however, in the case of indirect shots, there is an important cost factor because the sensors have to be changed periodically.

It is an element of initial monitoring and very useful in patients who do not tolerate intraoral procedures. It allows us to obtain important general information.

In the event of any type of finding, the decision must be made after a request for other types of radiological examinations. Digital panoramic radiography is an alternative and it uses lower doses of radiation with better image resolution.

Tomography

With digital tomography, a great advance has been generated in the diagnosis and planning of treatments. The images have the lowest distortion rate (between 0.2 and 0.5 mm). The interaction of this type of radiographic takes with other systems allows direct interaction in planning and clinical procedures in real-time.

Study Models

This is one of the oldest diagnostic methods in dentistry. It should always be presented articulated in a centric relation position and mounted on a semi-adjustable articulator.

In order to evaluate the occlusion, also possible premature contact points and compensation curves must be checked. If you don't use them, you may face treatment failure.

Digital prints

Intraoral scanners are based on different technologies but with the same objective: digitalizing dental preparations through cameras that capture images to generate a three-dimensional virtual model. The saved file has the extension STL (Stereo Lithography) and consists of a cloud of points joined by triangles.

Its main advantages are the comfort of the patients, immediate rendering of the patient's mouth digital models to analyze the dental preparation from different points of view and with magnification. And finally, it has a clean process.

Among its disadvantages, there is the learning curve, the use of opacity powder in most of them, the price of the hardware, and the limitations both in its indications and in the carvings.

Virtual Articulators

Just as in the production of prosthetic devices, working with articulators is the gold standard for dental laboratories, in order to ensure the same quality in virtual work, it is logical and consistent to maintain this standard in CAD-CAM systems.

Cerec offers an articulator function that offers us the possibility of determining both static and dynamic contact surfaces in order to improve or correct functional occlusion.

Through the software, we can observe the complete trajectory of the opening and closing movement. This tool is very useful since it allows us to eliminate premature contacts or interference at the occlusion level with just a click of the mouse.

Photographs

The importance of photography is that it allows us to document our clinical cases from the pretreatment, during the treatment and after the end of the treatment. In post-treatment, it allows us to publicize our cases through masterclasses, conferences, seminars and publications without neglecting legal defence or the identification of patients in legal or judicial processes.

Its advantage over analog is that we obtain the image and verify its exposure immediately, the possibility of editing, archiving on computers or storage devices and communication via email.

Cell phones are becoming more sophisticated since there are currently some that have between 10 to 12 MP of resolution featuring zoom adjustment, ISO or sensitivity, white balance among other options.

When taking extraoral photography, we must do it in the "natural position of the head", with the ears visible, without earrings or glasses; with appropriate lighting on the back of the patient to avoid shadows. The shots to be taken are **frontal**, strict **lateral** and **45º**, the three in rest position, maximum intercuspation, smile and forced smile.

For intraoral photography we must use a macro objective (ideally a 100mm or 105mm macro), a ring-flash to observe irregularities, color and texture of the enamel surface (the ring flash flattens the images), mirrors, separators and testers. The shots to be performed are frontal, right and left lateral, upper and lower occlusal, upper-whole area.

Planning wax-up

Here I am going to make an important suggestion. The planning wax-up is a physical projection of the result that we will obtain after the treatment of the patient is finished.

It is erroneously called diagnostic wax-up, because in Health Sciences the diagnosis is the identification of the disease and not the end result, so the diagnosis is made on models without any modification of cut or apposition by wax.

The planning wax-up will give us the guidelines for completion and the idea of proportionality between the teeth.

Diagnosis and Prognosis

We must define both terms before we can record them in clinical history and understand their importance in solving the case.

"Our future dictates the laws of today."
Nietzsche

We based on the vision of what we want to achieve, we analyze what we find, we diagnose and we plan. The diagnosis is the analysis that is carried out to determine any harmful situation and what are the trends.

This determination is made on the basis of systematically collected data and facts, which allow better judgment of what is going on. Here we must record the result of the study of all the alterations that we found in the evaluation and define the cause of the disease and the alteration of the function that our patient presents.

The prognosis is basically the prediction about the evolution of a patient's possible treatment, and the final result of the recovery process from the disease.

Treatment and Evolution Plan

It is important that we can establish not one, but several treatment alternatives. The primary step is the control of the immediate ailment, continuing with the simulation of the masticatory function, which is corrected through planning waxing.

Treatment alternatives allow the patient to choose which one suits their possibilities and what you are looking for so that based on this, we can establish the development plan of the treatment to be carried out. This section records the development of the treatment plan until its completion.

I hope to have achieved my mission with this chapter: to see how a correct medical history, with clear concepts, allows us to have treatments that drive to a successful recovery of our patients.

Before finishing this chapter, I am going to quote a Greek teacher, he spoke of what a judge should do, it was said more than 2,000 years ago but I think it fits perfectly with what we want to achieve with a medical history today:

"Listen politely, answer wisely, weigh wisely, and decide impartially."

This is **MIDAS TOUCH**. Welcome to the **ALPHAS**.

Dr BAK NGUYEN

CHAPTER 10

"PLANNING STRATEGY"

by Dr JULIO CESAR REYNAFARJE

Every time we are starting a new case, a new challenge begins. We must prepare ourselves to give it our best. Every patient is unique and reacts differently. That what's make it fun and interesting! Otherwise, we would be dying of boredom at our job.

10 years ago, I took charge of the treatment planning course at the university. I was always impressed that many highly skilled and knowledgeable students did not know how to organize their work, not only that, as the cases became more complicated, the margin of error was greater. That led me to generate a logic and a follow-up that allows us to plan any case.

As we are developing a **functional element** of any nature, it is important to have as much data as possible, organized and sorted to generate a **solution element**.

By sorting the elements, the order of the data obtained in the diagnosis is a decisive factor in the planning strategy. This ordering allows to be more efficient clinically, to be more effective and have better precision as we develop the planned phases.

This chapter will show us how to organize the data obtained for the diagnosis and to develop the stages of the treatment plan. But before starting a treatment plan, we must define the terms vital for our clinical case.

STRATEGY

A strategy is a plan to address an issue. A strategy is made up of a series of planned actions that will help you make decisions and achieve the best possible results. The strategy is aimed at achieving an objective following an action guideline. A strategy comprises a series of tactics that are more concrete measures to achieve one or more objectives.

Unifying concepts, a strategy is basically a group of rules that ensure a good decision at all times, and we can say that it differs from tactics. It is an ensemble of measurements and actions that allow the development of strategies to be put into practice.

The latter is a set of plans that must be carried out to achieve a goal. These strategies allow the creation of different plans that combined with tactics, allow the completion of the objective.

PLANNING

Planning is a method that allows executing plans directly, which will be carried out and supervised according to the strategy.

There are several ways to plan, but all of them have the same logic: forms, methods and actions are devised in order to achieve the goals set in the strategy, in an orderly and efficient manner.

There can always be unforeseen events that can jeopardize our planning, such as biological reactions that come from entities outside the treatment area, resistance to adaptation, resistance to technological changes or methodologies, and the lack of information in the strategic generation, all of which can bring the plan to a standstill or implement the plan in inappropriate ways.

STRUCTURING OF PLANNING STRATEGIES

Once the main terms are defined, we must generate a strategic work structure that allows us to add information as we develop our planning. Every case can have an array of different ways to achieve the same goal but they all have a specific logic order. We can understand that logic following matrix mesh.

In dentistry, in order to generate a strategy, we must face 4 main strategic axes in order to plan successfully:

- Initial prioritization Matrix
- Functionality Matrix
- Precision Matrix
- Matrix of Emotion

THE INITIAL PRIORITIZATION MATRIX

It is a diagram in which a series of signs of diseases are longitudinally related and confronted one to another. The idea is to **give a value to the importance of each disease**. Each sign its value. These values are defining which tasks are more important and will prioritize the sets in the treatment plan.

The first rule, before caring out the rehabilitation treatments, whether functional or aesthetic, we must eliminate the primary disease first. Usually, the diseases with the highest prevalence are those that have a bacterial or viral aetiology. A functional diseases will be prioritized as a second momentum.

Under this initial pattern, we must choose the procedures according to the speciality area and base our decision on the degree of importance and virulence. Conclusion? we have to clean the place first.

THE FUNCTIONALITY MATRIX

After cleaning the environment, you have to see how everything is working. When we talk about functionality, we are talking about the set of stomatognathic structures and the dynamic relationships that occur between them as part of the system, this being a set of functional elements that include teeth, joints and chewing muscles.

As mentioned earlier, after getting rid of the infectious origin, we must bring our attention to all the functional elements. But first, we must comprehend the logic and implication of each action (functional correction procedures); all the procedures work together, there are no functional elements completely independent. They all act as a system, a whole.

THE PRECISION MATRIX

Once our system works properly, we can now restore. For that, we must operate with precision. This is a necessary term in any dental procedure. It is based on dispersing the set of obtained values that are not close to the real value of the object or reference structure. The smaller the dispersion, the greater the precision.

The precision elements are all those that will be included in the functional pattern restored in the previous process. This matrix orders all the procedures with which we restore each and every one of the pieces of the dental arches and their supporting tissues.

THE MATRIX OF EMOTION

Finally, every clinical procedure involves an **emotional component** on the part of the patient. Technological advancements within the last 20 years have allowed patients to understand and foresee the scope and nature of their surgeries and procedures.

In simple words, they have expectations that we will have to manage. An aesthetic result, a painless procedure, the pace and the duration of the surgery…

Especially in aesthetic, the increasing knowledge of the patient generates, in many cases, a psychological and emotional imbalance. This is an important part of the whole problem that we will have to address.

The prioritization of dental aesthetic elements must be integrated into the facial pattern, allowing our rehabilitation procedures to be harmonious and reaching the patient's expectation.

PLANNING THE FLOWCHART

"It is believed that there is something called destiny,
but it is also believed that there is something else called will.
What qualifies man is the balance of that contradiction."
Chesterton

As dentists we will read it this way: instead of destiny we will say treatment success, and as the author says it is dependent on its will and balance.

Will is what allows us to choose the procedures, and the balance is based on the diagnosis and the judgment of the treating physician, this is how a planning flowchart is carried out.

Any procedure done in the mouth must be included in a prioritized procedures development plan. This will limit the surprises and complications. And, when encountered, will permit to manage effectively the emergency and/or complications.

Longitudinal monitoring is part of this approach and should be carried out following the sequence suggested in each phase of analysis and strategy.

TRANSFER SPLINTS

Transfer splints are clinical elements that allow the planned elements to be carried out in the mouth under the primary concept of precision, but with a basis of functionality and emotion already contemplated in the strategy.

Transfer splints can be of 2 types:

- Cutting splints.
- Adding splints.

Usually, the **cutting splints** are generated in the **Functionality phase** to be able to generate planes and the elimination of interferences. It is the first element of recovery of spaces in a functional relationship.

Adding splints are elements that **restore the morphology** and function of the dental elements included in the treatment plan.

In the next two chapters, we will spend some time on each of the phases of Strategic Analysis of clinical treatments.

"Everything we do has to be molded with the warmth
of our humanity, otherwise it does not make sense."
Dr Julio Cesar Reynafarje

This is **MIDAS TOUCH**. Welcome to the **ALPHAS**.

Dr BAK NGUYEN

CHAPTER 11

"PRIORITIZATION AND FUNCTIONALITY MATRIX"

by Dr JULIO CESAR REYNAFARJE

The development of the two topics of this chapter will allow us to understand the way to approach a treatment effectively, making it a success in its culmination.

Correctly ordering the logic of treatment is something that many times we do not get from school. We received a lot of knowledge, we achieved the ability to perform procedures, but to do, first requires a main factor: **experience**.

Logic allows us to generate an invisible sequence that analyzes several factors simultaneously and allows an order. That is the basis of a planning strategy.

The prioritization matrix, as already mentioned above, is the basis of the strategy, and the initial matrix is the basis of the other matrix, all the support of the treatment is carried out on the tissues previously prepared by this stage.

The functionality matrix, in turn, is the axis of movement, just as we do in aesthetics with the dynamic vision that overlaps the static one, the function must be preserved so that the rehabilitation elements behave correctly.

This chapter will allow us to make a correct conceptualization of our first strategic steps towards the development of our patient's treatment plan.

INITIAL PRIORITIZATION MATRIX

"Strong reasons make strong actions."
William Shakespeare

Dental planning is likewise. We have to reason and develop our ability to generate critical thinking that allows us to plan and then take actions in our treatment.

Often the complicated part of developing a treatment plan is not defining the type of treatment that the patient requires, the challenge is **prioritizing** the procedures.

It is important to recognize that not all the treatments that we establish initially have the same importance and impact on the clinical case. Some are the main point of the problem while others are only derivations of the former.

The difference between them leads us to a tool called prioritization matrix, which facilitates decision-making and obtaining solutions.

ROLE OF THE PRIORITIZATION MATRIX

In simple words, the prioritization matrix is a graph in which a series of evaluations relate and confront each one another. The important thing is that the information we obtain generates a quantifiable value in order to define which procedures are of more importance and guide the decision process.

All clinical cases are different, which is why each professional implements this tool according to their own needs. However, in broad strokes we can describe a series of functions associated with the prioritization matrix:

- Assess the evaluation criteria, as these are what tell us how relevant the planned procedures are. Without them, prioritization and classification processes would be impossible.
- Correctly define the type of diseases or clinical situations that in many cases we do not perceive with the clarity with which we should.
- Do an analysis of solutions or alternatives. Graph greatly helps to find solutions to problems and establish the execution plan.
- Always see opportunities for improvement. We do not always have to face a problem to look for alternatives. Improvement must be a constant element at any stage of any process.

| | | | | | | | | | INITIAL PRIORITIZATION MATRIX | |
Value	Condition	Surfaces	Value	Size of Cavity	Value	Pain	Value	Rx condition	Treatment Alternative	Priority
1	Caries	1	1	small	1	no pain	1	no	simple restoration	2
2	Crown Fracture	2	2	medium	2	low	2	sI	complex restoration	1
3	Periodontitis	3	3	large	3	medium			Inlay	1
0	vertical fracture/remanent	4	4	Pulpal condition	4	high			Onlay	1
		5							Overlay	1
									Corona	1
									Endodontics	3
									Post	1
									Extraction (0)	4
									Periodontal treatment	2
									periodontal surgery	2

An example of a priority matrix values.

BASIC STEPS FOR ITS APPLICATION

Now, let's move on to the practical zone. Do you know what are the essential steps for the implementation of the prioritization matrix, regardless of the type of case or its stages of execution?

Here I summarize them for you:

- Definition of diagnostic fields

Treatment plans use the prioritization matrix with one objective: to rank the individually diagnosed elements, facilitate decision-making, visualize problems, etc.

- Definition of the Options for the solution of the clinical case

Here the options are established to achieve the objective of the previous section. Sometimes they define themselves; others, however, must be established between the different types of treatments.

- Definition of the decision criteria

Also depending on the central objective, the professional must define the criteria to take into account. For example, if the idea is to rank the diagnosed conditions, some criteria could be the time of illness, the number of tissues affected, the degree of aggressiveness of the injury, etc.

- The weighting of criteria and options

Here the prioritization matrix is run for the first time. The different criteria are located in it (point 3) and compared with each other, assigning them a value that can be quantitative or qualitative. Immediately afterward the options are compared (point 2) by doing the same procedure.

- Select the best option

In the last evaluation, the criteria and the options are related. The value of each option is multiplied with that of each criterion and, finally, the option with the best score is chosen. That is the one that will be put in place to achieve the objective that we talked about in the first step.

The prioritization matrix are tools that help us organize a treatment plan, regardless of the need that prompts us to implement it. It is useful in any field or area of diagnosis and planning.

As applying the prioritization matrix in the planning strategy is the power of the professional, the choice is made according to the variables that are considered most important. The suggested variables are those of clinical assessment and number of treatments, but it can be more specific in prioritization using a larger number of variables in the evaluation phase.

After seeing so many numbers and possibilities, it is good not to forget that all this is to guide us through the process of doing things better; that within our humanity, the healing process must have the smallest possible margins of error.

The important thing is, before getting the patient on the dental chair, we have everything in order. In the case of complications, we could quickly react and adapt. That is the basis of planning, it is to act in the best interests of our patients.

When we start a treatment, by nature, we must control the infectious processes that appear to be able to generate a primary matrix. We use simple parameters of clinical evaluation and number of treatments, this allows us to order the process of healing the patient. The specialties that are usually included in this phase are:

- Surgery
- Periodontics
- Endodontics
- Restorative

All processes of infectious origin must be considered in this phase. In the case of surgery, problems such as the presence of root remnants, cysts, tumors, and non-dental elements included in the stomatology area are included.

When we talk about periodontics, the type of conditions to treat supra and infragingival stones, periodontal pockets, bone and gingival recessions with bacterial colonization varies. Gingival cuts for prosthetic or aesthetic purposes are not included in this phase.

In the case of problems that include the dentin-pulp complex, we are looking at endodontics, and reversible and irreversible pulpitis, pulp necrosis, problems in the periapical area such as cysts or purulent collections, are those that we usually classify in this phase.

Talking about restoratives we only consider lesions produced by caries disease that do not include the pulp chamber, usually, the restorations are functional and then be re-evaluated according to prosthetic and aesthetic points of view.

Multiple infectious elements may also be present as endo-perio problems, which can generate an element of higher priority assessment. This first matrix generates the first phase of treatments ordered to be considered in the treatment strategy and plan.

FUNCTIONALITY MATRIX

Once the primary problems have been eliminated, and if we want to say it with an example, after cleaning the device, we have to check it to see that it works well.

Always talk about the functional part in dentistry is associated with a complex element, let's analyze how to give it stability and make it simple.

Functionality depends on the relationship between the teeth of the upper arch with the lower arch when making contact at the time of closure. Dr Okeson complements this by saying that this occurs during jaw activity.

To make this matrix we have much more data to process, and first, we must generate a choice of the modifications in a staggered manner and following the natural process of evaluation.

The first thing to check will be the relationship between the anterior teeth, first check the overbite that is the superposition of the upper incisors on the lower incisors and is measured in percentage.

In second place, check the horizontal overjet or superposition of the upper incisors on the lower ones and is measured in millimeters. This is the first decision tool for the maintenance or adaptation of the functionality, and this is complementary to the comparison of facial thirds.

The second phase of evaluation is the inclination of the **occlusal plane**, for which we will take planes and cusps as reference. It is very important to define and maintain a plane, this should be made up of the incisal and occlusal surfaces of the teeth, taking into account the number of pieces present in the mouth.

If there were some missing, we would have to think about placing a temporary replacement such as a piece of wax, which Simulate the missing teeth in your arc position, arc shape, and offset curves.

In relation to the **Spee Curve**, an ideal imaginary line must be drawn that joins the buccal cusps of the posterior parts, which is convex for the upper jaw and concave for the lower jaw, which must coincide perfectly when entering the arches in occlusion, this line allows us to evaluate if we should make a cut or apposition on any tooth to allow a good functional movement.

EVALUACIÓN DE LA OCLUSIÓN				
Procedure	Clinical Value (1-5)	Complexity	Number of procedures	Priority
Vertical Dimension (Restoration)	3	1	6	18
Intermaxilary Relationship (Joint noises)	2	16	3	96
Oclusal planes (Interferences, extrusions)	2	32	3	192
Opening restrictions	3	1	1	3
Others	0		0	0
Total de Procedimientos			13	

FUNCIONALITY MATRIX

CLÍNICAL VALUES

Value	Description
1	chrónic asymptomatic
2	active asymptomátic
3	active with low symptomatology
4	active agresive asymptomatic
5	activo agresive with symptomatology

COMPLEXITY

Value	Description
1	Low
16	Medium
32	High

- Vertical Dimension (Restoration)
- Intermaxilary Relationship (Joint noises)
- Oclusal planes (Interferences, extrusions)
- Opening restrictions
- Others

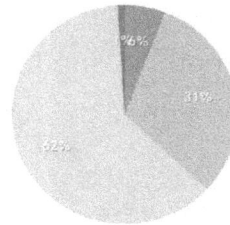

An example of how to make an easy Functionality Matrix.

Finally, we have the **Wilson Curve** that in a frontal view when drawing an imaginary line that passes through the buccal and linear cusps of the posterior pieces on both the right and left sides, a concave plane must be observed. This curve allows us to evaluate the anterior sector, and also to evaluate any cut or position in the sector.

Concluding the analysis, we are left to evaluate the laterality movements among which we have the canine guide and the group function, to be able to include cutting options to any interference in the function.

The protrusive movement is also evaluated and it is normal for the posterior pieces to become in occlusion, if there is contact in them they will be considered as interference.

We are now able to perfectly identify the priority position in our treatment plan of each element of urgency and functionality, we can already say that what we do will work on a patient who no longer has an oral or functional health problem.

Now, It's simple! Let's keep growing!

This is **MIDAS TOUCH**. Welcome to the **ALPHAS**.

Dr BAK NGUYEN

CHAPTER 12
"PRECISION AND EMOTION MATRIX"
by Dr JULIO CESAR REYNAFARJE

The Matrix systems that we are going to evaluate now are strongly related to each other. After generating patterns of release from infectious processes, and that the system meets the required parameters of functionality, we proceed to prosthetic rehabilitation, which must be carried out within **emotional patterns,** and also every procedure must be in **harmony** with the patient's physiology.

There are many cases in which we find restorations that do not go aesthetically with the patient's physiology and harmony, not even with the patient's sex since these restorations are made with incomplete information.

The purpose of including them with their own matrix is part of this effort of individualization and characterization following the **parameters of Sinestetics**, developed by Ahmad in his writings.

PRECISION MATRIX

We call them precision elements because every element that is a prosthetic restoration in the mouth must be exact, must adapt to the remaining surfaces, restore the missing areas and function.

All students, when they enter a postgraduate course, think that learning about new materials or new techniques is enough.

Taking these courses updates us on the trends, but we must learn to be able to apply them within our treatment plan.

In the case of materials, it is also necessary to act carefully, since no matter how good the function is, we can't always assume that it will always behave as expected. That's why we must always evaluate and apply them in a system, not only in a specific case.

When we classify the treatments, we have to be able not only to make a restoration of the affected pieces, but we also have to do the rehabilitation of the function of the stomatognathic apparatus, to achieve this we have to separate the treatment precision matrix into 3 primary areas:

- **Edentulous spaces area**
- **Restorations on Endodontically treated tooth**
- **Restitution of dental morphology**

We always do a secondary analysis with the prioritization matrix (Priority Planning) of this phase before deciding on the sequence, in addition to the choice of treatment there are two extra variables, the variable of **economic factor** and the variable of implantological factor.

EDENTULOUS SPACES AREA

When we talk about prosthetic restorations we can define it according to the parameters of oral rehabilitation, for this we could use 5 types of rehabilitation:

- Complete prosthesis
- Conventional removable partial prosthesis
- Removable partial prosthesis with attachments
- Fixed prosthesis
- Implant-supported prosthesis

Complete Prosthesis

It is a treatment considered from the moment the patient is totally edentulous, the evaluations are purely clinical and radiographic for the evaluation of possible remnants, this evaluation is carried out at the time of analysis and collection of information. It is a treatment that can be complemented by implantology, for better retention and function.

The prioritization of the treatment goes up in the matrix according to the number of missing pieces, you must consider the economic factor in planning to vary the treatment alternatives.

Conventional removable partial prosthesis

In the case of conventional removable partial prosthesis, it is an element of functional replacement of the missing pieces, it also has a social sense and improves the relationship life of the patient.

Partial prostheses usually support themselves from neighboring the edentulous sections, with retentive hooks that distribute the masticatory forces towards the support parts. For this reason, it is very important to achieve a good **balance of forces** at the time of distribution of these supports.

In the sequence of treatments, it is important to consider it as an alternative in patients without the possibility of rehabilitating implantologically, or with a fixed prosthesis. again, the economic factor variable generates several treatment options.

Removable partial prosthesis with attachments

Like the previous one, this alternative covers the edentulous gaps, restoring function, but this type of treatment has attachments included in crowns prepared in the parts neighboring the edentulous areas, this is a solution with higher retention than the previous one and eliminates visible retentive hooks making this a more aesthetic option than the previous one.

Fixed prosthesis

For rehabilitation with this type of procedure, we must prepare the pieces next to the eventual gap to be able to place a unique structure that we know as a prosthetic bridge that replaces all the missing pieces, including the 2 that were prepared. It is a second option after implantology.

Implant-supported prosthesis

Implant-supported prostheses are the best current alternative to rehabilitate the edentulous areas, this type of treatment allows us aesthetic and functional solutions with a better prognosis.

RESTORATIONS ON ENDODONTICALLY TREATED TOOTH

Endodontically treated tooth must be properly prepared in order to be functionally rehabilitated. All intra-root reinforcement must be supported by a dental remnant that allows the prosthetic restoration to be sealed over it. This must be done at the time of preparation, allowing the occlusal forces to be distributed throughout the dental surface implanted in the alveolar bed.

These procedures must be performed as a basis for the restoration of dental morphology.

DENTAL MORPHOLOGY

In this evaluation, we must consider all those procedures that restore the dental structure, its morphology and function in previously prepared pieces. Here we consider the single crowns, the aesthetic veneers and the restorations in composite. The ordering is done based on the priority of the precision area defined at the beginning and taking into account the trend of extra variables.

As we can see the recovery and restoration in the precision matrix depend on variables by indication of materials, analysis of occlusion forces, analysis of prosthetic support and finally the analysis of extra variables.

Believing that only through handling techniques and materials can we finish a case, can lead us to a greater error. To solve the patient's problem makes us responsible for them. It makes us love every day more what we do for them.

EMOTIONAL MATRIX

This is the final matrix, defines the individuality of the work to be carried out and allows our patients to have a rehabilitation according to its facial parameters, and integrates the smile into a functional and emotional framework.

The order of these factors also has **subjective parameters**, because we have the influence of the patient's opinion, but they can be framed according to measurable parameters on the patient's face, making it possible to generate patterns such as alignment and proportionality in addition to color patterns and texture, which are part of the aesthetic triad that must always be considered for this type of evaluation. Much of the subjective information is found in the **PPQ**, must be valued and quantified as done in the previous matrix.

" To be successful as in aesthetic dentistry,
one must be able to unite art to function."
Dr Julio Cesar Reynafarje

Aesthetics always will be a specialty in continuous evolution, and taking the words of Dr Pilkington is the art of making our work an inapparent improvement. To achieve this, we have to be able to **unite art to function** and this union is what is now called **Functional Aesthetics**.

When I started using this term in 2005 as the name of a post-graduate program, it was totally unusual, but time showed that they are intimately linked.

Now my concern is to be able to provide guides so that the aesthetic procedures included in our functional treatment are easy to perform, I hope to achieve my goal and serve you as much as it does in my daily work.

Before starting the analysis, it is important to take into account some basic aesthetic rules.

The first concept that we must be clear about is the so-called **Aesthetic Triad**. It is based on the Pilkington concept and is made up of the Shape, Texture and Color of our teeth, which can be valued and generates a prioritization.

The success of our aesthetic rehabilitation is based on these factors, missing one of these parameters automatically jeopardize the final result, the satisfaction of the patients and/or the stomatologic function.

PSICOMORPHOLOGIC EVALUATION				
Procedure	Clinical value	Complexity	Number of procedures	Priority
Facial	5	1	6	30
Dental morphology	4	16	3	192
Texture	2	1	3	6
Color	3	32	1	96
Sectorial	4	1	1	4
Other	0	0	0	0
Total Procedures			14	

CLÍNICAL VALUES

Value	Description
1	No distortion
2	distortion not measurable
3	Low Distortion (until 10%)
4	Moderate Distortion (10% to 30%)
5	Distortion (More than 30%)

COMPLEXITY

Value	Description
1	No distortion
16	distortion not measurable
32	Low Distortion (until 10%)

EMOTION MATRIX

● Facial ● Dental morphology ● Texture
● Color ● Sectorial ● Other

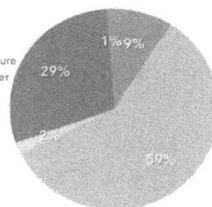

1% 9%
29%
2%
50%

Example of an Emotion matrix.

Therefore it is of uttermost importance to obtain harmonious aesthetic results. To do so, we must pay very close attention to these standards and the importance of the dental anatomy, color and textures to reproduce natural dental structures more naturally. The **best aesthetic surgeries are the ones people do not notice**!

When we start our treatment and based on the previous concepts, the factor that does not alter the usual function (which will be maintained or corrected during our treatment) is the color.

We must consider 2 procedures associated with color, which must be previously performed and stated in our treatment plan:

- Recording the Color of the natural teeth
- Bleaching procedures

Both procedures are recorded in this matrix but must be recorded in the treatment plan just after the execution of the first and second matrix, this allows making a correct choice of materials in precision and emotion matrix.

All these information are important guide in our daily work. They are just suggestions that optimize the quality and efficiency of our treatment plan.

I am sure that with this guide we are going to enjoy this often forgotten pleasure that is planning, and see a smile in our patients with our final result. That, for me, is the reward. This is our life!

"The Midas Touch is the confluence
of humanity and knowledge."
Dr Julio Cesar Reynafarje

This is **MIDAS TOUCH**. Welcome to the **ALPHAS**.

Caught between technological advancements and COVID 19,
our TOUCH will keep our relevancy.

Dr BAK NGUYEN

CHAPTER 13
"THE Y TURN"
by Dr BAK NGUYEN

Writing with Dean Reynafarje, I learned much, even after nearly 20 years in the profession. We are from different cultures, but above all, we share two different angles of the passion for dentistry.

I was forced into dentistry to respect the wish of my parents. I spent the last 20 years, finding ways to cope and to connect with my patients looking for human connexion. That was my beacon of hope. Strangely enough, that made my success in this dry world of science and medicine.

"I treat people, not teeth."
Dr Bak Nguyen

That philosophy made my career and my success. Coming from a completely different environment, Dean Reynafarje is in love with his profession. Going through his chapters, you can feel the passion of the procedures and matrix, the **WHY,** the **HOW** and **WHEN,** are not just protocols to him, they are more than science; with his love, he elevates them to the status of art.

But strangely enough, we both come to the same conclusion, to show our humanity through our art and craft. I believe that this is what it meant to be whole, to grow beyond our white coats. I elevated my craft and skill, looking for connexions and salvation. He did the same, from passion and dedication.

We can both say that we succeed in our careers as dentists. No dentist will serve as Dean of Education if not from the love of his profession, respected by his peers and colleagues. No entrepreneur can disrupt an entire industry if he wasn't successful and trustworthy.

Here we are, on the top of a profession that forged us into what we are. That's the white coat. We became successful the day we forged our white coat with our WILL and dedication. That's the humanity we brought on the table.

I gave you my experience and how I reached such a state. Julio did the same with his matrixes. With our combined views and techniques, you now possess the means to stir your profession beyond the white coat that you've received.

We started this book with the idea of easing your evolution in the profession, finding success and happiness. Well, this is the way, to grow your skill and craft with your humanity.

This is the Y turn, one looking to embrace and one looking to escape, we both arrived at the same crossroad and the path of success.

You can either hate your profession or be practicing your dream profession, it does not change your recipe to success, to find your humanity, and to build from, and with it.

As hard as it was for me to totally immerse myself into Julio's vision and matrix as I reviewed his chapter, I discovered a common passion, the commitment for the solution, the outcome. Be obsessed with your outcome, the one you gauge from the eyes of your patients and success is right around the corner!

This is the hope that you bring on the table, no matter your state of mind, your reflection in life, especially in the post-COVID era, you have a true shot to revive your passion through success, happiness and humanity.

This is our human touch, our Midas touch.

This is **MIDAS TOUCH**. Welcome to the **ALPHAS**.

Dr BAK NGUYEN

PART III
"MIDAS TOUCH"
Dr PAUL OUELLETTE

CHAPTER 14

"50 YEARS OF ABUNDANCE"

Dr PAUL OUELLETTE

My interest in dentistry started when I was a teenager at 13 years of age, in need of braces. My parents were not rich by any means. The cost of braces in those days was less than $1000, but not affordable for many families. Today multiply that number by five or six times.

Our family lived in a nice suburb in West Chicago called Oak Brook, Illinois. We had recently moved from St. Paul, Minnesota when my father started a packaging company he named Century Packaging. My father was one of the top leaders in packaging sales at 3M - Minnesota Mining and Manufacturing Company located in Saint Paul, Minnesota.

Family expenses were very heavy for my family after the move. Due to their financial situation at the time, they took me to a dental school in downtown Chicago for my orthodontic treatments. The original Loyola School of Dentistry established in 1923 was located in a very dangerous part of Chicago. The dental school was about a block or two away from Taylor Street, Home of the "Taylor Street Dukes".

Out of curiosity when writing this chapter, I researched online the history of Taylor Street Gangs in the 60s. I remember going to White's Saloon on Taylor Street with my co-dental students most every Friday after school. I was curious to see the history of the area 50 years ago.

I found the following information on Wikipedia:

THE TAYLOR STREET JOUSTERS

The Jousters, formally the Almighty Taylor Street Jousters, were a Chicago street gang that originally started on the Southside of Chicago and then later branched out to the north side of Chicago as well. Their name is a reference to the medieval sport of jousting. They later became part of the People Nation Multi-gang Alliance.

The Jousters started in the late 1960s, around the area of Ashland and Taylor streets, calling themselves the Taylor Street Jousters. The Taylor Street Jousters were an offshoot of a gang that previously controlled the area, that gang was known as The Taylor Street Dukes.

The ethnic makeup of the Taylor Street Dukes, and then later, the Taylor Street Jousters was primarily Italian.

During my trips to downtown Chicago to have my braces adjusted, we were able to park close to the school. We did not have to go into the surrounding neighborhood.

However, when I was accepted in Dental school at Loyola, after graduating from college at Texas A&M in 1966, dental students and medical residents had to park several blocks away from the medical centers.

That meant we all had to walk through the surrounding neighborhoods every morning and evening to get to and from our respective medical and dental schools.

One of the unspoken benefits of the neighborhood was any student enrolled in med or dental school had parking stickers on their cars related to Loyola, Presbyterian St. Luke's,

University of Illinois Medical School and Loyola Stritch School of Medicine.

With that sticker on, we were protected! We were the **CHICAGO UNTOUCHABLES**. We took care of the neighborhood's medical and dental healthcare and they took care of us.

THE GREAT CHICAGO BLIZZARD of 1967

One day, as I was in my first year of dental school, the GREAT CHICAGO BLIZZARD of 1967 struck northeast Illinois and northwest Indiana early morning on January 26-27, 1967. There was a record-setting two feet of snowfall in Chicago and its suburbs before the storm abated the next morning.

As of this writing, it remains the greatest snowfall in one storm in Chicago's history. The snow was just starting as I drove to dental school. Thankfully our dental professors closed the school and sent us all home around 10 AM.

The expressways were closed shortly after I made it back home. It took a week before we could resume school. Back in the day, a week seems like an eternity. Nowadays, in COVID time, a week is barely a breeze...

I will always remember how cold Chicago is even more so than St. Paul Minnesota, my previous home. Chicago is called the Windy City. The wind chill in downtown Chicago makes it one of the coldest places in the USA every year. Maybe that's the reason our family all moved to Florida.

My dental education was outstanding as we had many famous dental educators such as Harry Sicher, a world-renowned Anatomist, Dr Joseph Jarabak, Chairmen of Orthodontics and Dr Don Hilgers, PhD, Dr Jarabak's protege.

Dr Hilgers was the attending orthodontic resident under Dr Jarabak's supervision. I had the opportunity to learn about orthodontics from two of the masters. I finished my dental school education in 1970 and completed Dr Hilger's orthodontic program in 1972.

Immediately after graduation from my orthodontic residency, I moved to Atlanta, Georgia, to join my parents in a new vibrant southern city with no surprise blizzards. However, when Atlanta gets less than an inch of snowfall the whole city shuts down.

Southerners and snowbird transplants in the same city can not navigate the winding hilly streets of Atlanta during minor and moderate snowstorms. Atlanta was not far enough south for our family!

I spent my first three years post-graduation in Atlanta teaching orthodontics to residents and starting my first private practice. It was truly a wonderful experience. I joined the orthodontic faculty at Emory and married one of my patients, Patricia. We had three children together and I adopted her 6 year-old daughter, Cindy.

Patricia helped me develop over forty-five years together 33 orthodontic practices. She also raised and educated our children and together we created the "**Ouellette Family Dental Dynasty**". My full-time teaching position at Emory was for 3 years.

I had to resign to devote more time to our very successful practices. Pat and I, with our children's future contributions, had the Midas Touch. After 10 years in Atlanta, we sold all our offices and I retired early to sunny Florida.

For a year or more, we invested in Real Estate. Patricia and I found a beautiful riverfront one acre mini-estate on the Indian River in Eau Galle Florida. We paid $135k for a main house, 2 guest houses and a garage apartment. Then, we invested half a million in renovation costs. Patricia planned and oversaw a Victorian renovation of the four buildings.

We traveled to San Francisco frequently, taking pictures of the "Painted Ladies" Victorian houses. This is the style that made our renovation unique in the old Florida Cracker homes neighborhood.

THE WIKIPEDIA DEFINITION OF FLORIDA CRACKER

Architecture in a style of vernacular architecture typified by a wood-frame house. They built their homes surrounded by wide verandas or porches, often wrapping around the entire home, to provide shade for their windows and walls.

We were living our dreams! We added a lighted tennis court in the front yard and boat dock in the backyard on the Indian River. Patricia's inherited knowledge from her father who was in the construction industry as a mason. This background helped her serve as the general contractor for our new dream home project.

Patricia told me that she and her sister Jeanette used to carry buckets of stucco on job sites for their father. They learned a strong work ethic very early as I did from my 97-year old mother.

Patricia's father installed carpet, framed houses and had acquired most subcontractor skills over his 50-year career. This is how Patricia learned her design and building skills.

Pat's sister Jeanette became my first orthodontic assistant. She worked for 40 years in orthodontics. Her last employer was the world-famous multi-orthodontic practices developer, Dr Robert Pickron. He was also one of my mentors and taught me the business of orthodontics.

Patricia traveled back and forth from Atlanta shopping for architectural antiques that were incorporated into the four buildings. The home sold several years later to one of the auto dealership owners in Melbourne Florida for $2.6M.

Our two boys Jonathan and Jason were finishing their middle school education in Melbourne Florida. Melbourne and Cocoa Beach are two of the well-known surfing destinations in

Central Florida. Most of their friends would surf every day rather than concentrate on their homework and perform well in school.

Patricia and I discussed moving back to Atlanta for our kids to start in a new High School without the surfing and drug culture they were starting to be exposed to in Florida. My wife traveled to Atlanta and found a ranch home across the street from one of the best schools in Atlanta, Holy Innocents in Sandy Springs.

We paid $250K for our new 4 bedrooms home. The children could walk across the street to school. 3 years later, the school wanted to buy our home and the other three homes across the street on the main road Mt. Vernon Hwy. They also purchased several homes in another subdivision behind us to build a large soccer field and sports-related building.

An under the road tunnel was constructed to the athletic site across the street from the school where our front yard was. Patricia doubled our initial investment and found an estate home on 2 acres a mile from the school she purchased for $625K. She remodeled the new home's basement and a few rooms upstairs at first.

Then she said we will never be happy with a home with 8-foot ceilings. She hired an architect to design a 12,000 square foot home on the two acres estate lot. The original home was about 5000 square feet, came with a lighted tennis court and in-ground pool.

Patricia removed the 5000 home and, in two years, constructed a 9 bedroom, 12 bathroom, 6 fireplaces, added an indoor lap pool, gym, wine cellar, a stadium seated home theater under the 3 car garage, resurfaced the tennis court, constructed a pool house and outbuilding a garden building. Our estate was magnificent.

We hosted several charity events for our children's school and other organizations. Our family was living the American Dream!

We were offered $4.5M for our home, but we did not want to sell at the time. Our daughter Danielle had two more years of high school and she did not want to leave her newly made friends. Our sons had graduated from high school and were starting their College educations.

Patricia and I were hoping our children would join the Ouellette Family Dental Dynasty. Of course, both boys wanted to do anything but dentistry at first. Our family's hard work, community service, and wonderful-blessed lifestyle was definitely influential and motivated our children to match and surpass our accomplishments. They finally wanted to live the American Dream as Dental Specialists.

Initially, Jason chose to pursue a career in economics and finance at the University of Georgia. He graduated with a finance degree from the University of Georgia's business school.

He was immediately recruited by a very successful mortgage company in Atlanta. He learned to package and close home loans during the real estate boom. He routinely had more than 40 active files at a time that would yield him $2000 or more at each closing.

That was until a real estate bust-recession hit the mortgage industry in the year 2000. Being laid off by his new employer was a life-changing opportunity for him. He FINALLY decided to join the family's business. He enrolled at Georgia State University and commuted by MARTA transit to the downtown Atlanta campus to take the required pre-dental course.

Three years later he graduated with a chemistry degree and applied to Dental School. He was accepted to University of Pacific, in San Francisco.

UOP had an accelerated three-year dental school program. It was one of the best programs in the country at the time. There were many famous dental educators that taught Jason and influenced him to pursue orthodontics like his father. Dr Robert Boyd was the chairman of Orthodontics.

Dr Boyd is an orthodontist and periodontist. Bob took Jason under his wing and helped him for the three years when he was at UOP. Dr Boyd is the original researcher who helped develop digital dentistry solutions such as clear aligner therapy. He and his orthodontic department performed most of the early clinical research and development of the Invisalign system.

Our family will always be indebted to Dr Bob Boyd, Professor Emeritus. Bob is currently Director of Digital Technology and Solutions at Aligntech, San Jose California.

Jonathan bounced around enrolling in two or more colleges. He was always very talented in computer programming and loved video games. Jonathan had a keen interest in creating music and composing soundtracks on his Macintosh computer using a program called Protools.

Jonathan moved back to Florida and enrolled in a computer music program at Full Sail University in Orlando Florida. He spent his next two years learning how to create music in a professional studio setting.

Upon graduation, he came back to Atlanta and joined the team at Zac Studios in downtown Atlanta. He loved all night sessions working with famous recording artists that traveled from Nashville to Atlanta to record in Zac's 7000 square foot $5 million equipped studios.

He loved working with the 3 recording studio's high-tech sound-recording consoles. Zac Studio is now called Astro Studios and still in Atlanta under new ownership since 2017.

FROM SOUND ROCKSTAR TO DENTAL IMPLANT DRAGON

My son, Dr Jonathan, took the circuitous path to become a dentist. Now becoming a sound engineer he decided to open his own studio in Atlanta. Guess who Bank rode the venture?

After a few years, he finally decided that being happy as an artist wasn't going to pay the bills forever. As fate would happen, our family was invited to our cousins' wedding in Miami Florida. He was marrying a beautiful girl from Bogota, Columbia.

The wedding was to be held in a waterfront mansion located on Star Island, Miami, very close to the homes of Julio Iglesias and Rosie O'Donnell. Our family traveled from Atlanta to Miami on a Thursday.

I had to stay until Friday evening as I was busy with my multiple practices in Atlanta. When I checked in the hotel Friday evening, no one was around as they all were night coming after the rehearsal party.

The next morning I asked where my son Jonathan was hanging out? Everyone said we haven't seen him since he met a beautiful Columbiana girl named Tania at the rehearsal dinner. I did not see Jonathan and his new Colombian girlfriend until the ceremony.

Tania came from a very prominent family in Bogota. She and her family were living the Colombian dream with multiple servants and bodyguards, with bulletproof limousine transportation due to Drug Cartels' kidnapping problem in Colombia.

Tania was the architect and studied abroad in Spain and England. She was very beautiful and sophisticated. Jonathan was invited to visit her in Bogota. When he returned home he wanted to move to Colombia.

At the time the country was still under siege with violent-related incidents being the norm. Groups such as the Revolutionary Armed Forces of Colombia (FARC), National Liberation Army (AUC), 19th of April Movement (M19) and the Medellin Cartel still active and kidnapping was a major problem.

You can imagine how my wife and I, felt about Jonathan's new living quarters in the middle of the Cartel related terrorist groups and drug wars. Tania assured us that it would be safe for Jonathan to visit Colombia and attend school at Pontifical Xavierian University, aka Javeriana University.

Jonathan moved to Columbia to start his new adventure. In his first week in Bogota, Tania said this is the last time we will speak in English in this house! She enrolled Jonathan at Javeriana University's "total immersion" Spanish Course. In six months he became moderately fluent in his new language and was able to pass the medical admissions test that was given totally in Spanish!

It was ironic that his best new male friend in his program came from a Spanish-speaking family. Matthew was taking the same Spanish course to improve his grammar. He and Matt sat for the medical school entrance examination together. Jonathan passed on his first try and his friend Matt had to wait six months to retake the exam.

Matt later finished all his required medical school courses, residencies and is now a plastic surgeon in Augusta Georgia. Matt's mother is on the Medical College of Georgia's Dental Faculty.

Tania learned the business from her parents and is quite a talented businesswoman. When she was studying architecture. She and her girlfriend started a part-time business manufacturing exotic scented soaps. Their part-time business turned into a booming network of standalone stores in the "Zona Tay" in the upscale areas of Bogota.

On one of our visits to see them, we stayed in a hotel in Bogota. In our room's bathroom were the Lotto Brand soaps created by Tania. She also had business interests in Cartagena and was in most of the major Hotels in this Colombian seaside city. Tania's new condominium was on the high side of a mountain overlooking the beautiful city of Bogota.

Most people do not realize that Bogota is at an elevation of 8660 feet situated in the Andes Mountain range making it one of the highest capital cities of the world. It is always cool in the evenings (45°) and warms up to about 65° during the day.

If you look at a mobile phone weather app, the temperature in Bogota and San Francisco is almost the same every day. The weather is absolutely spectacular in Bogota. There is usually no need for air-conditioning when living in this beautiful city. Maybe a little heat in the evenings helps. When I grow up I may move back down there.

Dental education in Columbia is usually a five-year program. Right out of high school, you enroll in a dental emphasized college program. Your first year is studying basics like most USA colleges. After your first year, you then start dental school training.

This worked out great for Jonathan as he already had been exposed to basics in the USA. He concentrated on learning his Spanish skills during his first year. Halfway through Jonathan's first year in the medical school program, he decided he may have made the wrong choice.

He went to the director of the medical program and said he would like to see about transferring into the dental school program. She took Jonathan over to the director of the demo program.

This was just going to be a quick introductory meeting and Jonathan will schedule an appointment to talk with her. As fate would have it, she unexpectedly had time to meet with Jonathan that day.

More than three hours later, he comes out of the room and was admitted to the dental school program starting the next week. Jonathan said that he really hit it off with the director and they talked more about the why he moved to Columbia and was going to be the first-ever gringo dental student in the history of the University.

My wife Patricia and I traveled many times down to visit Jonathan in Bogota. We also invited our good friends of 40 years, Dr Pete and Jade Pickron to come with us. We met all of Jonathan's instructors and professors. Dr Pickron and I presented on numerous occasions lectures about Orthodontics, Orthognathic Surgery and Practice Management.

Jonathan became a rockstar in Bogota! The majority of dental students in Colombian dental schools are at the bottom of the prestige polls. The only gringo to study dentistry at Javerianna had lockers in the Oral Surgery and Periodontist Clinics. Jonathan attended many of their clothes treatment planning meetings after hours.

He was asked to translate Journal articles and book chapters into English by his teachers and dental colleagues. When my wife and I would spend a week or more in Bogota, Jonathan's faculty and dental specialty colleagues would invite us to their parties.

At every party, the doctors and their spouses wanted to hear Jonathan's story. My wife and I had to excuse ourselves to go get another glass of wine and spend time in the kitchen with the cooks and servers.

Most of Jonathan's teachers spoke fluent English, but it was easier for Jonathan to tell his story in his new native tongue. This was repeated often at all future parties as they were all so fascinated with his story.

We were invited on weekends to their summer Villas in the mountains and or their Fincas (Farms) to ride horses. We all learned about a new beautiful culture. Our family has considered eventually retiring in Colombia if the Cartel Wars end one day.

Jonathan completed his studies over a period of seven years. He returned to the USA and enrolled in the University of Florida in the UF AEGD advanced dental training course. The two-year course is a prerequisite for being able to sit for a USA state board of dentistry examination.

In Jonathan's last year at the University of Florida, he was recruited by Dr Michael McCracken, Prosthodontist and Dr Guy Rosensteil, Implant Dentist and Sedation Instructor to become the Lutheran Medical Sponsored program Chief resident at the Foundry Charity Medical Center in Bessemer, Alabama.

Jonathan completed the one year program at the foundry and started his dental practice in the Orlando area of Florida. He purchased a small declining practice and medical building in Altamonte Springs, Florida.

The practice owner was in his last five years of practice. Practice revenues were declining as he only focused on hygiene services and referred most procedures out to other doctors. At the time of purchase, his revenues were only going to be about $175,000 for the year.

Jonathan took over the practice and within three months he had added that much production on the books as he knew how to do the majority of procedures that were previously sent out by the selling doctor.

At that time Jonathan upgraded the equipment in his practice adding 3D CBCT Imaging, Cerec intraoral scanning and a same day crowns mill plus other needed upgrades.

At the end of his first six months and years-end, he had produced more than $500,000 in dentistry. The next year it was easy for him to collect $1,000,000. Today, Jonathan is known as the IMPLANT DRAGON.

I am proud of my sons as they are both following our long-standing family business plan and legacy to provide affordable high-quality dentistry.

THE NOW

Jason is the Director of Orthodontics at Dr Joel David and associates in Jacksonville Florida. Dr David invented the D5 ultra teeth in 24-hour system. The D5 system provides a permanent hybrid dentures solution versus most other providers only deliver a plastic or PMMA or plastic denture. It then takes another 8 to 9 months or to have the permanent hybrid denture fabricated out of a Zirconia permanent material. Jonathan is Dr David's Central Florida D5 provider.

Last year Jonathan delivered 128 full arch hybrid dentures supported by 6 dental implants. The procedure is like the All-on-Four System, but the D5 Ultra Teeth adds two additional implants in case of future implant failure. In case of implants failure the denture may have to be remade. This is less likely to happen with Dr David's game-changing invention.

I am in my last 5 to 10 years of active patient care. I currently am working for a DSO producing more than $3 million a year out of three offices in Atlanta, Georgia. It's hard to believe at my age of 76, that it is still possible to produce that much dentistry.

With the help of a good dental management team, it will be possible to continue at that pace. However, I am moving my practice to a virtual cloud-based model. My Pakistani and USA web-developers and I are developing a software application that will allow me to see patients from my iPhone, mobile tablet or laptop computer.

I am seeking consulting partnerships with dentists and dental specialists to treat orthodontic and dental implant patients. The TADplant provisional dental implant will be hopefully approved by the FDA by year's end. The TADplant is a Pediatric or Temporary dental implant that was designed over the last 10 years to solve a long-standing problem.

Most pediatric patients are thought to be too young for dental implants. Implant dentists have historically avoided placing dental implants in an 11-year-old child. The **TADplant** was designed like a **TAD**, aka Temporary Anchorage Device. Orthodontists and dentists have been placing **TAD**s for more than 25 years.

A **TAD** is a temporary dental implant that is used for orthodontic "anchorage". That is a **TAD** implant stands firmly in the bone and will not move when forces are applied from the **TAD** to a tooth or group of teeth. **TAD**s can be placed in less than a minute and removed months or years later in less than 30 seconds.

The **TAD** implant does not affect the implant receptor site and it may actually preserve bone due to micro-vibrations during functional forces such as chewing and breathing. I used the same concepts in designing the **TADplant**, a two-piece temporary dental implant, that will support a temporary or even a permanent crown to stimulate the implant receptor site preserving bone and hopefully preventing need for a future bone grafting.

I knew virtual practice will support dentists and orthodontists that are performing adjunctive orthodontics and **TADplant** provisional implant dentistry. I am looking forward to working with my younger colleagues and avoiding hands-on aerosol producing procedures at my age.

We have discussed the **BEGINNING** and the **NOW** of The Ouellette Family of Dentists - Dental Dynasty. The future is bright for the family. There will be ups and downs. We can handle them with the help of our colleagues.

Our dental practices are beginning to re-open after the CV-19 Pandemic. The Future of Dentistry has changed forever. There will be new innovations that will maintain and improve the safe delivery of our services.

Dentists have historically provided patient-safe dentistry even before the current pandemic. It was AIDS 30 years ago, SARS, Ebola and Zika several years later that mandated all dentists provide CDC, ADA, state dental board and national professional association ordered patient protective sterilization protocols.

We are just going to do more of the same best practices with added changes to protocols that we learned from the current CV-19 Pandemic and the next pathogen pandemics coming at us.

Life is GOOD NOW and will be REALLY GREAT in the NEAR FUTURE.

This is **MIDAS TOUCH**. Welcome to the **ALPHAS**.

Dr BAK NGUYEN

CHAPTER 15

"THE JOURNEY"
by Dr BAK NGUYEN

From the beginning of **THE ALPHAS**, I had the privilege to meet with Dr Paul Ouellette, our **ALPHA DEAN**, with not only 50 years of dentistry under his belt, but laying the foundation of a dynasty of dentists.

Both Julio and I insisted for Dr O, Paul Ouellette, to join this book and share with us his journey of 50 years. Talk with the man for more than 10 minutes and you soon realize how profoundly happy and fulfilled Dr O is.

At 76, he is still talking about future projects, not just traveling and enjoying, but about the future of dentistry, of a new way to replenish our profession and new dental technologies to develop. Some, he is presently developing.

There are 2 generations of dentists between Paul and I, but we get along as we were brothers. Actually, that's how he calls me, a brother from another mother!

No one can undergo 50 years of profession and still be that enthusiastic about it if it wasn't a great ride! Surely, Paul found the Midas touch in dentistry. From humble origins, he managed to elevate himself to the rank of doctor in dental medicine, then, of specialist in orthodontic and professor of orthodontic.

In our previous book together, **RELEVANCY**, Paul shared with us the how and the details. But, in this installment, he shares his story, from where he started, and also his broader story, the one beyond his white coat.

From his debut as a student to the path of a millionaire, Paul always walks the dental path. Even his wife, he met on the dental chair. Together, they found happiness and success.

Paul is very open with us on his journey, sharing the numbers and how he rose from a dangerous neighborhood to the millionaire districts of two different states. This should give hope to anyone of us, looking for more from our journey.

He made it and did not impose his recipe on his children. They went their way and chose their own path. "Two of our three children, after different career paths, joined the family dynasty of dentistry." Isn't that the dream of many parents? Of most of us? Not only to succeed but to be happy and to stretch that success and happiness to the next generation?

Well, that's the hope that Paul Ouellette is bringing on the table, not bragging but sharing with all of us his journey and anecdotes.

We each have our unique style and unique experience. Each of us has reach success wearing our white coat. Paul did that for 50 years and is looking ahead for many more to come.

On that, I will join my friend Julio to say how beautiful our profession is, we just need to find our way to navigate it. I know, reading Paul's words was a surprise to any of you. I was surprised myself, looking for dental words.

Well, that's the humanity he brought to our white coat, to go beyond it! Is that a working recipe? He successfully inspired a second generation of dentists within his ranks. Look at his friends, they aren't just dentists, they are the pioneers of our profession on more than one front.

I am privileged to have Paul as a friend and brother from another mother.

We do not have to be perfect. We do not have to be alike. We just need to be respectful and open to the uniqueness and difference of each other. The sensitivity that we allow ourselves is the first sign of kindness that our patients will identify and bond with.

We do not want to impose on anyone since imposing is the worse sign of insecurity. We are doctors, our role is to serve and to heal. Why not take the opportunity to inspire too?

This is what Dr Paul Ouellette is doing, inspiring each and every one of us to let go and to explore our full potential, leaving the restrictions and limitations behind. He went above and beyond what was expected of him. He did so without a revolution nor challenging the entire world. He did it with kindness and a light touch.

That's the Midas touch, Paul Ouellette's touch!

This is **MIDAS TOUCH**. Welcome to the **ALPHAS**.

Caught between technologic advancements and COVID-19,
our TOUCH will keep our relevancy.

Dr BAK NGUYEN

CONCLUSION
by Dr JULIO CESAR REYNAFARJE

The country where I live has a diversity of nuances and spectacular landscapes. From immense deserts to unexplored jungles, with giant mountains that look at the horizon with passivity and majestic, which make every trip to any place an adventure.

Near these mountains, you will see rivers of crystalline waters born from the Andes that sprout from the earth to unite with the rain, connecting all this diversity of colors and scents of impressive naturalness that fill all the corners of the land of my birth.

These rivers when they form, make their own channel. It is very difficult to change. Nature guides them on their way to the sea. Why I am telling you this? Because I feel that this book, is like one of these wonderful rivers that follow their destiny. Bak, Paul and I just let flow what we think, feel and live, making **MIDAS TOUCH** a book that flows from life, mind and heart.

When we talk about life, Dr Paul Ouellette leads us honestly, wisely and humbly through a story of growth, where the dreams of one person become the reality of an entire family.

History of work, of love for what you do, demonstrates the profile of an academical trained professional with success within his specialty that knows no border: his life's experience, the professional careers of his children, and today, his influence over many new dentists, each of which, have their unique vision of the future. His journey and story reflect the quality of the person that he is.

Talking about what we think is sometimes complicated, especially when it comes to dentistry. Being in medical science, all information must be verified with research. We are facts based, research is the resource on which science is based to continue growing. It is the basis for the development of new technics and technologies to improve the treatment of our patients.

Prior to the admission of a dentist in a clinic, he or she has to learn protocols and standards of treatment. Nevertheless, each patient is a new challenge, a unique challenge, because not only do you need to have knowledge but you also need to have criteria too.

That was my challenge in these chapters, ordering the criteria. The way we think while seeing a patient must be an easy and understandable way for the general dentist, the specialist, and the patient. That should be easy for everyone to understand and follow. That way of thinking makes our work more predictable and increase our chances of success of both parties, doctor and patient.

Talking about feelings and mindset in dentistry is a topic very little addressed in our field. I must say that Dr Bak Nguyen does it with mastery and with incredible eloquence. Bak is a born innovator, he develops and explains what is the feeling of a person dedicated to this medical career.

Dr Bak not only understands the way a dentist feels but chapter after chapter, he is shaping a successful mindset within the profession, empowering through its own experience the reader, to live and to look forward with the hope of improving and helping our society to feel better.

Finally, as Rainer Maria Rilke said, "Works of art are always born from those who have faced danger, from those who have gone to the extreme of the experience, to the point where no human can exceed.

The more you see,
The more your own,
The more personal,
The more unique
Life becomes.

The work we do leads us to make our life a mixture of passion, knowledge, experience and love, which leads us to make into works of art everything we touch, every day of our lives, for the good of our patients, with a Midas touch.

This is **MIDAS TOUCH**. Welcome to the **ALPHAS**.

Dr BAK NGUYEN

ABOUT THE AUTHORS

From Canada, **Dr Bak Nguyen**, Nominee EY Entrepreneur of the year, Grand Homage LYS DIVERSITY, and LinkedIn & TownHall Achiever of the year. Dr Bak is a cosmetic dentist, CEO and founder of Mdex & Co. His company is revolutionizing the dental field. Speaker and motivator, he wrote more than 72 books in 36 months, accumulating many world records (to be officialized).

From Peru: **Dr Julio Reynafarje**, dentist, Dean of the Peruvian Dental Association postgraduate School of continuing Education. Postgraduate professor for more than 15 years, with more than 100 international lectures and with publications in many languages in magazines worldwide, he is also the author of the book Sfumato in Esthetic dentistry and is an active entrepreneur in Medical issues.

From USA: **Dr Paul Ouellette**, DDS, MS, ABO, AFAAID, WORLD TOP 100 DENTISTS, Former Associate Professor Georgia School of Orthodontics and Jacksonville University. A visionary man looking for the future of our profession.

UAX

ULTIMATE AUDIO EXPERIENCE

A new way to learn and enjoy Audiobooks. Made to be entertaining while keeping the self-educational value of a book, UAX will appeal to both auditive and visual people. UAX is the blockbuster of the Audiobooks.

UAX will cover most of Dr Bak's books, and is now negotiating to bring more authors and more titles to the UAX concept. Now streaming on Spotify, Apple Music and available for download on all major music platforms. Give it a try today!

www.DrBakNguyen.com

AMAZON - APPLE BOOKS - KINDLE - SPOTIFY - APPLE MUSIC

FROM THE SAME AUTHOR
Dr Bak Nguyen

www.DrBakNguyen.com

THE POWER OF YES 5 074
VOLUME FIVE: ALPHA
BY Dr BAK NGUYEN

THE POWER OF YES 6 075
VOLUME SIX: PERSPECTIVE
BY Dr BAK NGUYEN

www.DrBakNguyen.com

AMAZON - APPLE BOOKS - KINDLE - SPOTIFY - APPLE MUSIC

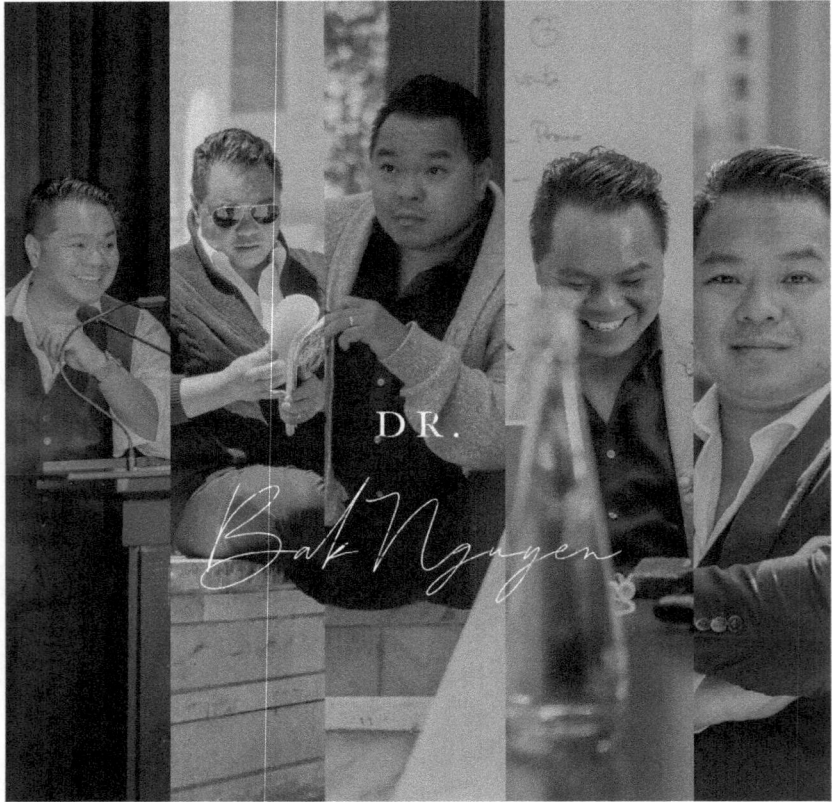

DR.

Bak Nguyen

www.DrBakNguyen.com

www.ingramcontent.com/pod-product-compliance
Lightning Source LLC
Chambersburg PA
CBHW061216220326
41599CB00025B/4661